"It has long been recognized that health care does not follow the rules of free markets, yet the United States continues to rely on a dysfunctional financing system that fails to correct for these market deficiencies. In *Health Care Wars*, John Geyman shows us how this has been a disaster, while providing us hope through the prospect of empowerment of patients and taxpayers."

—Don McCanne, M.D., Senior Health Policy Fellow,
Physicians for a National Health Program (PNHP)

"*Health Care Wars* debunks the propoganda served up by self-serving commercial interests. Author John Geyman blows away the smokescreen hiding the profit motives of health-care related entities. He diagnoses the disorders inherent in the present health care non-system. This book imagines a humanitarian health care system unsullied by profit motives and guided by scientific evidence."

—Joseph S. Silverman, M.D., Distinguished Life Fellow,
American Psychiatric Association

HOW THE SECOND GILDED AGE IMPACTS AMERICAN FAMILIES

"It's no use pretending that what has obviously happened has not in fact happened. The upper 1 percent of Americans are now taking in nearly a quarter of the nation's income every year. In terms of wealth rather than income, the top 1 percent control 40 percent. Their lot in life has improved considerably. Twenty-five years ago, the corresponding figures were 12 percent and 33 percent. One response might be to celebrate the ingenuity and drive that brought good fortune to these people, and to contend that a rising tide lifts all boats. That response would be misguided. While the top 1 percent have seen their incomes rise by 18 percent over the last decade, those in the middle have actually seen their incomes fall."

—Joseph E. Stiglitz, Nobel laureate in economics and former chief economist at the World Bank.[1]

1. Stiglitz, JE. Of the 1%, by the 1%, for the 1%. *Vanity Fair*, May 2011.

"Most American families are worse off today than they were three decades ago. The Great Recession [now continuing] of 2008-2009 destroyed the value of their homes, undermined their savings, and too often left them without jobs. But even before the Great Recession began, most Americans had gained little from the economic expansion that began almost three decades before. Today, the Great Recession notwithstanding, the U.S.. economy is far larger than it was in 1980. But where has all the wealth gone? Mostly to the very top. . . . The rapid trend toward inequality in America marks a significant reversal of the move toward income equality that began in the early part of the twentieth century and culminated during the middle decades of the century."

—Robert B. Reich, professor of public policy, University of California Berkeley and former U.S. Secretary of Labor in the Clinton Administration[2]

2. Reich, RB. Foreward to Wilkinson, R, Pickett, K. *The Spirit Level: Why Greater Equality Makes Societies Stronger*. New York. Bloomsbury Press, 2009. p. ix.

HOW HEALTH CARE MARKETS FAIL PATIENTS

1. Predatory pricing
2. Perverse incentives for profit
3. Consolidation and market power
4. Inefficiency and bureaucracy
5. Inadequate quality control
6. Volatility and unreliability
7. Unethical practices
8. Outright fraud

HOW THE U.S.. NOW 'LEADS' THE WORLD IN INCOME INEQUALITY, HEALTH AND SOCIAL PROBLEMS

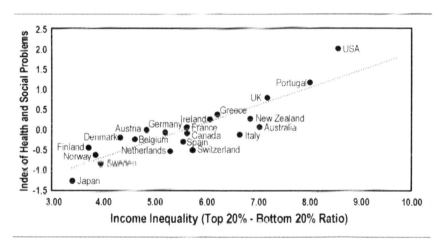

The more unequal countries are in income distribution, the higher the numbers of health and social problems.

Source: Reprinted with permission from Wilkinson, R, Pickett, K. *The Spirit Level: Why Greater Equality Makes Societies Stronger*. New York. Bloomsbury Press, 2009, p. 174.

THE "WISDOM" OF THE MARKET

"In a free market, the system of prices is the emergent result of a vast number of voluntary transactions, rather than of political decrees as in a controlled market. The freer the market, the more truly the prices will reflect consumer habits and demands, and the more valuable the information in these prices are to all players in the economy. Through free competition between vendors for the provision of products and services, prices tend to decrease, and quality tends to increase. A free market is not to be confused with a perfect market where individuals have perfect information and there is perfect competition.

Free market economics is closely associated with laissez-faire economic philosophy, which advocates approximating this condition in the real world by mostly confining government intervention in economic matters to regulating against force and fraud among market participants."
—Wikipedia. Free market. (http://en.wikipedia.org/wiki/Free_market, accessed January 24, 2012

"Conservatives for Patients' Rights (CPR), established in 2009, describes itself on its website as a "non-profit organization dedicated to educating and informing the public about the principles of patients' rights and, in doing so, advancing the debate over health care reform . . . Any serious discussion of health care reform that does not include choice, competition, accountability and responsibility—the four 'pillars of patients' rights—will result in our government truly becoming a 'nanny-state,' making decisions based on what is best for society and government rather than individuals deciding what is best for each of us."
—Website for Conservatives for Patients' Rights, accessed October 5, 2009.

"Our survey of national health insurance in countries around the world provides convincing evidence that government control of health care usually makes citizens worse off. When health care is made free at the point of consumption, rationing by waiting is inevitable. Government control of the health care system makes the rationing problem worse as governments attempt to slow the use of services by limiting access to modern medical technology. Under government management, both efficiency and quality of patient care steadily deteriorates."

[We conclude that]:

"1. The competitive private health care marketplace is more efficient and provides greater value than government-financed health care.
2. Health care costs can be contained if overuse is managed by giving consumers more choice and responsibility for their own health care decisions.
3. The more technology, the better the health care.
4. We don't ration care as much as do countries with national health insurance.
5. National health insurance is socialized medicine.
6. The American public is too individualistic to want national health insurance."

—2002 report by the Dallas-based National Center for Policy Analysis, a conservative think tank established in 1984, with excerpts from Geyman, JP. Myths and memes about single-payer health insurance in the United States: A rebuttal to conservative claims. *Intl J Health Services* 35 (1): 63-90, 2005.

"Able-bodied adults should save enough on a regular basis so that they can provide for their own retirement, and for that matter, health and medical needs."

—Paul O'Neil, as Secretary of the Treasury in 2001 and former top executive at two large multinational corporations, as quoted by Hartmann, T, *Unequal protection: The rise of corporate dominance and the theft of human rights*. Emmaus, PA. Rodale Press, 2002, p. 177-8.

"I don't want to abolish government. I simply want to reduce it to the size where I can drag it into the bathroom and drown it in the bathtub."

—Grover Norquist, lobbyist and president of Americans for Tax Reform, as quoted on NPR's Morning Edition in May 2001.

"Health plans are leveraging technology to improve systems that result in greater efficiencies and improved care. We are working with doctors, pharmacists and others to build secure systems to safeguard important medical data that can give patients the option of quickly and securely providing their medical history to a new doctor. Innovative partnerships with academic institutions are promoting patient safety by warning doctors, pharmacists and patients about harmful prescription drug interactions. These are just two of many innovations that health plans and their partners are working on to improve health and our health care system."

—Home website of America's Health Insurance Plans (AHIP), accessed on January 24, 2012. (http://ahip.org/Driving-Innovations/)

"Healthcare spending on the dual eligible population [Medicare and Medicaid] is estimated at more than $300 billion annually, with managed care plans serving just a tiny portion.

But that's about to change as states increasingly turn to health plans to help control costs. All of which spells huge opportunity for insurers in need of growth. . . . We expect to have representatives from leading Medicaid and Medicare plans, federal and state governments, and the Wall Street and investment community in attendance. It's an opportunity you won't want to miss."

—Attention Health Plans Seeking Growth: How Does $300 Billion in New Business Sound? Invitation to a Managed Healthcare Forum by the Corporate Research Group on The Dual Eligible Opportunity for Health Plans, to be held on April 18, 2012.

"Single-payer health insurance differs from many private insurance companies in one important respect—no profit motive. But, far from [stockholders] being a burden, having no stockholders removes any incentive to operate efficiently. In fact, national health insurance provides all the wrong incentives for both the health care system and the patients in the system."

—Goodman, JC, Herrick, DM. Twenty Myths about Single-Payer Health Insurance: International Evidence on the Effects of National Health Insurance in Countries Around the World. National Center for Policy Analysis. Dallas, TX, 2002, pp. 38, 64.

Also By John Geyman, M.D.

The Modern Family Doctor and Changing Medical Practice

Family Practice: Foundation of Changing Health Care

*Family Practice: An International Perspective in Developed Countries
(Co-Editor)*

Evidence-Based Clinical Practice: Concepts and Approaches (Co-Editor)

Textbook of Rural Medicine (Co-Editor)

Health Care in America: Can Our Ailing System Be Healed?

*The Corporate Transformation of Health Care:
Can the Public Interest Still Be Served?*

Falling Through the Safety Net: Americans Without Health Insurance

Shredding the Social Contract: The Privatization of Medicare

The Corrosion of Medicine: Can the Profession Reclaim its Moral Legacy?

*Do Not Resuscitate: Why the Health Insurance Industry is Dying,
and How We Must Replace It*

*Hijacked: The Road to Single Payer in the Aftermath of
Stolen Health Care Reform*

*Breaking Point: How the Primary Care Crisis
Endangers the Lives of Americans*

*The Cancer Generation: Baby Boomers Facing a Perfect Storm
Second Edition*

HEALTH CARE WARS

How Market Ideology and Corporate Power are Killing Americans

John Geyman, M.D.

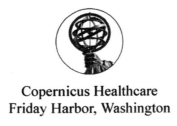

Copernicus Healthcare
Friday Harbor, Washington

Health Care Wars: How Market Ideology and Corporate Power are Killing Americans

John Geyman, M.D.

Copernicus Healthcare
Friday Harbor, WA

First Edition
Copyright ©2012 by John Geyman, M.D. All rights reserved

Book design, cover and illustrations by W. Bruce Conway
Cover photo courtesy of iStockPhoto
Author photo by Anne Sherridan

softcover: ISBN 978-0-9837734-8-1
eBook: ISBN 978-0-9837734-9-8

Library of Congress Cataloging-in-Publication Data
is available from publisher on request.

Copernicus Healthcare 615 Harrison Street #D,
Friday Harbor, WA 98250

www.copernicus-healthcare.org
john@copernicus-healthcare.org

Dedication

To Gene, with thanks for all your support and encouragement over these 56 years. You are the love of my life and soul mate. I dedicate this book to you.

And for the:
- 50,000 plus Americans who die each year for lack of health insurance
- the 50 million uninsured and growing tens of millions of underinsured Americans who struggle to gain access to basic health care
- the 2 million cancer patients who forgo recommended care due to unaffordable costs
- the 2 million Americans who go bankrupt each year due to health care costs
- U.S. employers who want coverage for their employees but can no longer afford it
- physicians and other health professionals laboring in the trenches of health care under an increasingly burdensome private sector bureaucracy that steals time from care of their patients
- taxpayers who pay more and get less from our market-based system driven by profits for the private sector
- legislators and policy makers who bear responsibility for our current problems and become part of the solution.

May we all see a better way that protects our children and later generations from the havoc of failed market policies in U.S. health care.

Contents

PART I
Health Care Markets: A Failed Experiment

PART II
How Health Care Markets Fail—And Can Kill You!

PART III
Beyond Market Failure—What Can We Expect?

TABLES AND FIGURES

Acknowledgements

I am indebted to these colleagues for their constructive comments and suggestions through their peer review of selected chapters:

- Allan S. Brett, M.D., Professor and Vice Chairman of the Department of Medicine at the University of South Carolina, Columbia
- Howard Brody, M.D. Ph.D. Director of the Institute for the Medical Humanities, University of Texas Medical Branch, Galveston
- Richard Deyo, M.D., MPH, Kaiser Permanente Professor of Evidence-Based Family Medicine, Oregon Health and Science University, Portland
- Joshua Freeman, M.D., Professor and Chairman, Department of Family Medicine, University of Kansas Medical Center, Kansas City, KS
- David Gimlett, M.D., long-time family physician and former Medical Director of Inter Island Medical Center, Friday Harbor, WA
- Larry Green, M.D., Epperson-Zorn Chair for Innovation in Family Medicine at the University of Colorado School of Medicine, Denver
- Don McCanne, M.D., past president of Physicians for a National Health Program (PNHP) and PNHP Senior Health Policy Fellow
- Charles North, M.D., professor of family and community medicine, University of New Mexico, Albuquerque
- Ted Phillips, M.D., professor emeritus of family medicine, University of Washington, Seattle
- Roger Rosenblatt, M.D., MPH, professor of family medicine, University of Washington, Seattle
- John Saultz, M.D., Professor and Chairman, Department of Family Medicine, Oregon Health Sciences University, Portland
- Rob Stone, M.D., emergency medicine physician in a community hospital in Bloomington, IN and Director of Hoosiers for a Commonsense Health Plan

Greg Bates, publisher at Common Courage Press, made many helpful editorial suggestions along the way, including those related to organization and direction of the manuscript and book design. After working with him as editor for this and six previous books, I continue to highly value his insightful suggestions. I am further indebted to Malcolm Sparrow, Ph.D., professor of practice of public management at Harvard University, for his guidance toward helpful resources concerning health care fraud; to Ralph Nader, J.D. and Joe Silverman, M.D. for their encouraging comments on the manuscript, and to Matt Wuerker, Khalil Bendib, Joe Heller, Jim Morin, and Rob Tornoe for graciously allowing me to reprint their excellent political cartoons.

Thanks are due to many investigative journalists, health professionals and others for their probing reports concerning our failing health care "system." I have found the work of many organizations useful in assembling an evidence-based picture of how our medical-industrial complex actually works in practice, especially reports from the Centers for Medicare and Medicaid Services (CMS), the Center for National Health Program Studies, the Center for Studying Health System Change, the Commonwealth Fund, the Congressional Budget Office (CBO), the General Accounting Office (GAO), the Organization for Economic Cooperation and Development (OECD), Public Citizen's Health Research Group, the Robert Graham Center for Policy Studies in Family Medicine and Primary Care, the U.S. Census Bureau, and the World Health Organization (WHO).

Special thanks are due to Bruce Conway, my associate at Copernicus Healthcare, who has been closely involved with this entire project from start to finish, ranging from book design of the interior and cover to preparation of graphics, typesetting, and conversion to ebook format. Mark Almberg of PNHP lent his experienced proof reading eye, and Carolyn Acheson of Edmonds, WA created a reader-friendly index for the book.

As always, I am most indebted to Gene, my lovely wife of 56 years, for her support and understanding over these many years, even as she gracefully dealt with declining health from Alzheimer's disease and sadly passed away shortly before this book went to press.

PREFACE

Market Failure: The Inconvenient Truth In U.S. Health Care

We have been told from time immemorial in this country that free markets, unfettered by government interference, are the fix for any of our problems. The notion that a competitive private marketplace gives us more innovation, choice, efficiency and value has been repeated so often for so long that it has become a meme (a self-replicating idea that is perpetuated regardless of its merits). Although this idea has become as American as apple pie and might work in some sectors of the economy, it does not work that way in health care. In fact, as this book will show, the private deregulated health care marketplace serves corporate stakeholders rather than patients and families, is unsustainable in its present form, and completely fails the public interest.

Today's market-based health care system is pricing itself beyond the reach of much of the population. Greed, profiteering and the business "ethic" are making even basic health care inaccessible to many millions of Americans even as politicians on both sides of the aisle avoid confronting the basic problems. In the same way that we have developed a military-industrial complex, despite President Dwight D. Eisenhower's warning in the 1950s, we now have an enormous medical-industrial complex that is powerful enough to fend off almost all efforts to rein in its abuses.

We are in the midst of an undeclared class war in this country that has only recently broken out into the open as something that we recognize and talk about. The shared prosperity that followed World War II gave rise to the American dream that brought new hope and opportunities for much of our population. But over the last 30 years, under a relentless attack by conservatives and willing Democrats, this dream is disappearing. As Joseph Stiglitz, Nobel laureate in economics, has observed: "Instead of a dream, we now have an American nightmare: a government of the top 1 percent, by the top 1 percent and for the top 1 percent."[1]

Unfortunately, this all too familiar list shows how serious the disconnect between the haves and have nots has become in our society:[2,3]

- The top 1 percent take in almost a quarter of the nation's income and control 40 percent of its wealth;
- Since 1970, the income of the top 0.1 percent of the population has gone up by an astounding 385 percent while the income of the bottom 90 percent of us has dropped by 1 percent;
- Based on a definition of the middle class as those between the 30th and 70th percentiles by income, one-third of Americans have dropped out of the middle class since 1980;
- Wages for the 70 percent of Americans without a college education have fallen precipitously since 1970 while corporate CEOs walk away with huge incomes, bonuses, stock options, and retirement packages even when they were considered failures.
- 25 million Americans cannot get full-time work, manufacturing has declined sharply, higher-paying jobs have been cut or outsourced overseas, leaving lower-paying service jobs here;
- One in six Americans falls below the federal poverty level ($11,170 for an individual and $28,820 for a family of four in 2012);
- 50 million have no health insurance, with tens of millions more so underinsured that their "coverage" is in name only;
- According to the annual Milliman Medical Index, the total cost of health care in 2011 was $19,393 (not a typo!) for a family of four in an employer-sponsored PPO, already a hardship level for many families, since the median household income for American families is about $50,000 [4]
- Not being able to afford care, a rapidly growing number of Americans delay or forgo necessary care, leading to higher mortality and worse outcomes down the line.
- As home foreclosures climb, a marked increase has also occurred for emergency room visits, hospitalizations and suicide attempts.[5]
- Despite all this bad news on the home front, the U.S. has also been slipping abroad—we are no longer the most competitive economy in the world, ranking fifth by a 2011 report of the World Economic Forum behind Switzerland, Singapore, Sweden, and Finland. [6]
- Meanwhile, the Centers for Medicare and Medicaid Services (CMS) project that national health expenditures, as a percentage

of GDP, will increase from 17.7 percent today to 19.8 percent in 2020 ($13,708 per capita) [7]

Henry Giroux, author of a new book *Education and the Crisis of Public Values: Challenging the Assault on Teachers, Students and Public Education*, has this to say about these big changes over the last 30 years:

"As the left slid into organizing around mostly single-issue movements since the 1980s, the right moved in a different direction, mobilizing a range of educational forces and wider cultural apparatus as a way of addressing broader ideas that appealed to a wider public and issues that resonated with their everyday lives. Tax reform, the role of government, the crisis of education, family values and the economy, to name a few issues, were wrenched out of their progressive legacy and inserted into a context defined by values of the free market, an unbridled notion of freedom and individualism and a growing hatred for the social contract." [8]

As the middle class withers away and as pensions, retirement plans, and safety net programs continue to erode, public confidence in government and the political process has reached it lowest ebb. The vast majority of Americans now believe that the democratic process has been handed over to ruling corporations and the political elite, with the U.S. Supreme Court anointing this change by allowing unlimited amounts of corporate money into politics.

Why this book now, and why isn't it being written by an economist? To the first question, it seems clear that these are darkening times, and the current political discourse as the 2011-12 election campaign heats up gives no sign for optimism about real reform. Copernicus Healthcare has moved to a rapid turnaround of a completed book (both print and ebook). So I hope that this book can help to educate the voting public and policymakers before the election is over.

To the second question, almost all economists still seem wedded to the myth of free health care markets, they themselves have not worked within the system, and the dry numbers of whatever they write tends to miss the human tragedy. I have had the opportunity to experience the changing health care system from the inside over the last 50 years, whether in rural family practice, in medical education, or in research and writing about the system.

We are in a time when the class war raging in this country is over the soul and humanity of America, over the future of the middle class, over what kind of a country we are, and over whether the American dream can be recaptured. These are more than economic issues—they are also social, political and moral issues. It will take an informed and activist voting public to counteract the power and money of corporate forces of the few and push our political leaders to responsible action.

Within the overall class war, health care wars are being fought on many fronts—ranging from the role of government in financing and policy making to whether contraception should be readily available to American women to whether or not the 2010 Affordable Care Act is constitutional. These wars cannot be won without winning the class war through a functioning democracy.

And why this particular subject for this book? My previous ten books on the health care system have peeled off one layer of the onion after another. But I have come to the conclusion that the single most important factor responsible for our runaway, unaccountable system is the free market concept that lies at its core. Other advanced countries around the world recognized this problem many years ago, and have controlled market abuses by various kinds of government oversight and regulation. As we head for the cliff, we need to wake up soon!

This book takes an evidence-based approach to assess and describe the track record of health care markets as they actually work. As you will see, it is a story of profiteering, greed and waste with very little accountability. I hope that this book is useful in informing the public, policymakers and politicians of the real problems with markets. We will need a strong and powerful unified grassroots movement to push our leaders toward real reform. The alternative to such action is dire—increasing odds of a national catastrophe and bankruptcies over health care, which can be prevented by mobilizing action plans as advocated in my last two books.[9,10]

John Geyman, M.D.
Friday Harbor, WA
April, 2012

References

1. Stiglitz, J. as quoted in Borosage, RL, Vanden Heuvel, K. The American dream: can a movement save it? *The Nation* 293: 15, 11, 2011.
2. Ibid # 1.
3. Rothschild, M. Enlist for class warfare. *The Progressive*, September 20, 2011.
4. Milliman. 2011 Milliman Medical Index, May 2011.
5. Kalita, SM. Tying health problems to rise in home foreclosures. *Wall Street Journal*, August 31, 2011: D1.
6. Saltmarsh, M. U.S. slips to fifth place on competitiveness list. *New York Times*, September 8, 2011: B9.
7. Office of the Actuary, Centers for Medicare and Medicaid Services. *Health Affairs*, July 28, 2011.
8. Giroux, HA. Corporate media and Larry Summers team up to gut public education: Beyond education for illiteracy, vulgarity and a culture of cruelty. *Truthout*, September 17, 2011.
9. Geyman, JP. *Hijacked! The Road to Single Payer in the Aftermath of Stolen Health Care Reform*. Monroe, ME. Common Courage Press, 2010.
10. Geyman, JP. *Breaking Point: How the Primary Care Crisis Endangers the Lives of Americans*. Friday Harbor, WA. Copernicus Healthcare, 2011.

PART I

HEALTH CARE MARKETS:
A FAILED EXPERIMENT

"Right-wingers, insurance companies, and other opponents of health care reform in the United States are always looking for ways to blame the government for the failures of our health care system. But the simple truth is that they have it backwards: our problems with health care are firmly rooted in the private sector. That is why the average high-income country—where government is vastly more involved in health care—spends half as much per person on health care as we do, and has better health outcomes."

—Mark Weisbrot, co-director of the Center for Economic and
Policy Research[1]

1. Weisbrot, M. Problems of U.S. health care are rooted in the private sector, despite right-wing claims. *McClatchy-Tribune Information Services*, July 20, 2011

"Far too much of American history is a history of greed—for land, furs, minerals, slaves, factories, art, power, recognition, and money without limits. Yet many of us want to believe that America is about something more and that our common effort can lead to a common good, not just the piling up of the latest plutocrats' privileges. Not all eras are defined by greed. For the first 30 years after World War II, for example, greed for a time seemed muted.[2]"

—Richard Parker, lecturer in public policy at Harvard's Kennedy School of Government and author of *The Myth of the Middle Class*[2]

2. Parker, R as cited in his review of Jeff Madrick's book *Age of Greed: The Triumph of Finance and the Decline of America, 1970 to the Present. The American Prospect* 22 (6): 61, 2011.

CHAPTER 1

Plundering Plutocrats: A 30-Year Undeclared Class War In America

"The true friend of property, the true conservative, is he who insists that property shall be the servant and not the master of the commonwealth... The citizens of the United States must effectively control the mighty commercial forces which they have called into being."[1]

— Teddy Roosevelt

"It has become difficult not to recognize that we are firmly in the grip of a second Gilded Age. Not only is this return obvious in the homage – if not hysteria – that marks a return to the dream worlds of consumption, commodification and survival-of-the-fittest ethic, but also in the actions of right-wing politicians who want to initiate policies that take the country back to the late 19th century – a time in which the reforms of the New Deal, the Great Society and the Progressive Era did not exist."[2]

—Henry A. Giroux, professor of english and cultural studies at McMaster University, Hamilton, Ontario, and author of *Politics After Hope: Obama and the Crisis of Youth, Race and Democracy.*

Across a rapidly expanding body of literature tracing the downward slide of America and the hollowing out of our middle class, there seems to be a consensus among writers that its most recent cycle started about 30 years ago. With the election of Ronald Reagan as president in 1980, the country made a sharp turn to the right, and is now in the midst of a class war pitting the affluent elite against the middle class and poor.

Some even identify the exact date when this war of ideas started. In his 2011 article "30 Years Ago Today: The Middle Class Died," Michael Moore makes the case that the middle class died on August 5, 1981, when the newly elected president fired every member of the air controllers union (PATCO) two days after they went on strike, further declaring their union illegal. PATCO had been one of only three unions that had supported Reagan for president. Remarkably, there was virtually no opposition to this bold action—the AFL-CIO, the biggest union in the country, even told its members to cross the picket lines, as did other unions, rapidly breaking the strike. As Moore observes: [That was the time that] "Big Business and the Right Wing decided to go for it—to see if they could actually destroy the middle class so that they could become richer themselves." [3]

Our country finds itself in a dire predicament today, in health care, education, manufacturing, household indebtedness, and untenable social and income inequality. Based on our current circumstances, we are forced to admit that Corporate America, so far, is winning this war. In order to more effectively counter these market forces and regain some semblance of the American Dream, we need to recognize how the battle has been fought by the right.

This chapter has two goals: (1) to sketch out eight key strategies by which the right has implanted its "values" at the center of political discourse and national policy today; and (2) to briefly describe the battlefield resulting from this war as it relates to possibilities and directions for health care reform.

Here we consider these eight strategies used by the right over these last 30 years:

1. Privatize everything to the maximum.
2. Throw Labor under the bus: outsource labor and dismantle collective bargaining.
3. Unleash the tiger: evade or prevent government regulation.
4. Be the message: control information and the media.
5. Be the government: infiltrate and take over much of the work of government.
6. Buy politicians: give campaign cash to make them yours.
7. Freeload: avoid corporate taxation as much as possible.
8. Rig justice: make use of a conservative U.S. Supreme Court.

Most readers are aware that these weapons are being deployed. But the details are surprising—and unsettling.

In the front matter at the beginning of this book, we laid out the major beliefs and assertions of the right concerning how markets are *supposed* to work. Classic "trickle down" economics, by which a rising tide is theoretically supposed to lift all boats. But it is now obvious that this is not true. Only the boats of the most affluent have risen. For the 99 percent, most of us have seen stagnation or loss of income as social and economic inequality have reached historic proportions.

THE CORPORATE COUP IN AMERICA: 8 KEY WEAPONS IN ITS CLASS WAR AGAINST THE MIDDLE CLASS

1. Privatize everything to the maximum.

With the brazen largely unproven claim that—private is better by bringing us more efficiencies and greater value—the right has succeeded in privatizing a large swath across our society and economy over the last three decades. These examples illustrate the breadth of their reach: finance, insurance and real estate (FIRE), health care (e.g. Medicare, Medicaid, hospitals, nursing homes, hospice, physical therapy), information management, prisons and water. Efforts to rip services out of the hands of government and privatize them, usually with a downgrade in services and higher costs, are rarely blocked. The most notable exception is Social Security, an effort withdrawn during the George W. Bush presidency.

The move toward privatization was aided by enabling trade agreements in the much-vaunted global economy. International agreements such as the General Agreement on Trade in Services (GATS) and the North American Free Trade Agreement (NAFTA) allowed multi-national corporations to gain expanded markets while outsourcing U.S. jobs overseas, thereby cutting their labor costs, avoiding the burden of employee benefits, increasing their profits, and sidestepping domestic scrutiny.

An enormous area undergoing privatization, which is still below the radar screen for most of us, is the notion of "competitive sourcing." In this way, much of the work of government is contracted out to private bidders, usually at prices much higher than if government itself did the work. In her excellent 2009 book *Shadow Elite: How the World's New Power Brokers Undermine Democracy, Government, and the Free Market,* Janine Wedel, a social anthropologist at George Mason

University's School of Public Policy, describes how government agencies are now forced to justify why they have *not* contracted out services to private vendors. Thus large corporations such as KBR, Halliburton, Blackwater, Raytheon and Lockheed Martin can amass huge profits while providing largely routine services for the government.[4] This is the same government that the right keeps wanting to cut down to size!

One of the problems of the larger role of private contractors in government work is the loss of control and accountability that it so frequently entails. An example of this is a 25-year contract awarded in 2002 for a joint venture of Lockheed Martin and Northrop Grumman to upgrade the U.S. Coast Guard. The Inspector General of the Department of Homeland Security later questioned the government's influence and involvement in the project, leading to an article in the *Wall Street Journal* entitled "Is the U.S. Government 'Outsourcing Its Brain'?" [5]

2. Throw Labor under the bus: outsource labor and dismantle collective bargaining.

Outsourcing of U.S. jobs overseas has accelerated in recent years beyond what most of us realize. We all know that much of our manufacturing has declined, together with a number of other industries, such as textiles. We also know that many call center and credit card transactions are based offshore. But white-collar jobs are also moving overseas at an increasing rate, ranging from such occupations as radiology, law, finance, and information management to clinical trial management and book editing.[6] A 2008 study by the Harvard Business School found that as many as 42 percent of U.S. jobs are vulnerable to be sent overseas.[7] As Arianna Huffington notes in her excellent recent book *Third World America: How Our Politicians Are Abandoning the Middle Class and Betraying the American Dream:* "Do you hear that? It's Ross Perot's giant sucking sound being cranked up to a deafening roar—and it's about more than NAFTA."[8]

As all this has gone on, the labor movement in this country has been decimated. Two examples serve as bookends for this trend over the last 30 years—Reagan's wiping out PATCO in 1981 and Wisconsin Governor Scott Walker's assault on collective bargaining in 2011. Union membership in this country has declined precipitously over the last three decades. After reaching its post WW II peak of 35 percent of the U.S. labor force in the 1950s, union strength continued to decline as jobs disappeared in many sectors of the economy. By 2009, just 12 percent of the workforce belonged to unions. In 2010, the Bureau of Labor Statistics reported a 10 percent drop in private sector union membership for the previous year, the largest single-year decline in more than 25 years.[9]

3. Unleash the tiger: evade or prevent government regulation.

The right maintains a continuing drumbeat of rhetoric claiming that the marketplace is perfectly able to regulate itself, and that too much interference by government will kill jobs and hamper innovation. Meanwhile corporate America has many methods at its disposal to weaken or avoid regulation by government. These range from lobbying politicians and placing their own industry representatives inside regulatory agencies to drafting the fine print of regulations in legislators' committees, moving some of their operations overseas, and clouding the issues with disinformation. One current example of the latter is the campaign now being waged by the U.S. Chamber of Commerce for "regulatory reform" (i.e. eliminating bothersome regulations). The Chamber proselytizes with snake oil declaring, for example, that regulations jeopardize American jobs and cost too much. The Coalition for Public Safeguards, which includes Public Citizen, has exposed the untruth of these disingenuous claims on its website www.chambersnakeoilfour.org.[10]

We all know of many examples of revolving doors between industry and government, but may be less aware of how sophisticated that effort has become. Wedel introduces us to the world of "flexnians," whom she describes as those who carry the "revolving door" to a new level—the *evolving door*." They are government-appointed insiders who craft policies with their own private purposes in mind, reorganize relationships between bureaucracy and business, and exert official power without public oversight. They become skilled at showing only a public persona that best meets their needs while obscuring their real agenda. One example given by Wedel is Steven Kelman, a Harvard professor in the Kennedy School of Government, who through a number of posts deregulated the very process of awarding government contracts. In 2007, he wrote an Op-Ed for *The Washington Post* railing against Inspector General reports as "generally advocating more checks and controls." At the same time he had an equity interest and served on the board of directors of a government contractor that the IG had recommended be debarred from receiving government contracts. [11-13]

We have only to look at some recent examples of regulatory ineffectiveness to see how much oversight by government has been eviscerated in this country—Enron, the Massey mine explosion, the massive Madoff fraud case, the BP oil disaster, and the Wall Street crash that put 8 million Americans out of work and set off a global recession, to recall just a few. Conflicts of interest abound across the corporate-government interface. As Paul Krugman observes about the cozy relationship between regulators and Wall Street:

"Wall Street is a huge source of campaign donations, and agencies that are supposed to regulate banks often end up serving them instead, but officials have also argued that letting banks off the hook serves the interests of the economy as a whole.[14]

James K. Galbraith, well-known economist and author of *Created Unequal: The Crisis in American Pay* and *The Predator State*, gives us this overview of what has happened:

[The corporate republic] has "turned over the regulatory apparatus to the regulated industries... the henhouse to the foxes in every single case. And that is the source of the abandonment of environmental responsibility, the source of the collapse of consumer protection, and the source of the collapse of the financial system. They all trace back to a common root, which is the failure to maintain a public sector that works in the public interest, that provides discipline and standards, a framework within which the private sector can operate and compete. That's been abandoned."[15]

4. Be the message: control information and the media. Over the last 30 years, the right has bought up and controls much of the media and the public discourse. To be fair, there are some exceptions, such as the *Huffington Post* and its linkage with AOL. The new media landscape ranges across television, cable-news networks, newspapers, magazines, the Internet, radio, book publishers, and well-funded conservative think tanks. The public is mostly unaware of the unseen hand of corporate control of many of these outlets. As an example, the ownership grip of now discredited Murdoch's News Corp. includes Fox News and the *Wall Street Journal*. Beyond ownership, interlocking directorates bind media together in ways that we could not expect to know. Thus, a 2009 study by Fairness and Accuracy in Reporting (FAIR) found that, among the nine major media corporations and their major outlets, six of the nine had board connections with pharmaceutical companies while there were board connections to six different insurance companies.[16]

Corporate interests have many ways to control and bias information delivered to the public in any of these media. To take one example, as reported by *The Nation's* Eric Alterman, Murdoch "regularly uses book deals, television contracts and columnist gigs as bribes to the powerful, just as he uses these same properties to punish those who refuse to go along."[17]

A recent report by the non-partisan Center for Budget and Policy Priorities has found that the major causes of the 2011 federal deficit were, in order:

- the economic downturn (e.g. less economic activity leads to less tax revenue and higher social service costs) (28 percent)
- the Bush tax cuts (40 percent of which went to those with annual incomes more than $500,000) (24 percent)
- and the wars in Iraq and Afghanistan (14 percent).

Yet a study by FAIR of the 69 nightly news segments in which the budget deficit was discussed during the first six months of 2011 found that only three mentioned any of these three leading causes of the deficit. In three-quarters of the segments, no cause was mentioned, while 12 identified misleading or inaccurate causes (such as Medicare and Social Security, which have nothing to do with the current deficit).[18]

Occupy Wall Street gives us another example of restricted and biased coverage. Coverage was delayed at the beginning, is still underreported, and tends to misrepresent protesters as not representative of a broad movement.

5. Be the government: infiltrate and take over much of the work of government.

As a result of an accelerating trend over the last two decades, incredible as it may seem, more than three-quarters of the work of the federal government (as measured by the number of jobs) is now carried out under contracts with the private sector.[19] These may take place under various kinds of mixed state-private entities, including "quasi-government" organizations (which may even include certain venture capital funds) and federal advisory committees that provide guidance to more than 50 government agencies.[20] This shadow government has even led to a new language—the word "governance" now substitutes for "government."[21]

The opportunity to govern is now being auctioned off to the highest bidder. The striking feature is that this practice has strong bipartisan support. As reported by *The Washington Spectator*, prices for key slots on congressional committees on both sides of the aisle are for sale and the prices are posted.[22]

This example reveals how far the current situation has departed from the democracy we still claim to have. The American Legislative Exchange Council (ALEC) is a powerful group completely funded by corporate interests that pursues this mission: "to advance the Jeffersonian principles of free markets, limited government, federalism, and individual liberty, through a nonpartisan public-private partnership." Beyond that rhetoric, here is how it operates. As exposed by a Democratic member of the Wisconsin State Assembly and reported in a 2011 issue of *The Progressive*, the organization is really a dating service between legislators and corporate special interests, matching them up, building relationships and promoting corporate-friendly legislation. Its 2011 annual meeting had about 2,000 attendees, about 40-50 percent legislators and 50-60 percent corporate and right-wing interests. They have task force meetings at their meetings to actually create model legislation in such areas as tax policy and health care. They vote on these task forces on these bills (with corporate members having the majority), then give advice on how to get the bills through Congress. Their intended policies, of course, include no new taxes, vouchers and block grants for health care.[23] According to the Center for Responsive Politics, PhRMA is the biggest spender on lobbying of the federal government on ALEC's Private Enterprise Board.[24] ALEC is also active in creating cookie cutter legislation, written by ALEC and sponsored by members of the legislature for action at the state level.[25]

6. *Buy politicians: give campaign cash to make them yours.*

The power of money in politics increased exponentially with the January 2010 U.S. Supreme Court decision (*Citizens United v. Federal Election Commission*) that allows corporations, unions and issue advocacy organizations to spend unlimited amounts of money, without immediate or complete disclosure of their sources, to influence political campaigns. There are a number of ways by which money is used to sway the electorate and influence public policy issues, including campaign contributions to candidates, election cycle ads, distribution of literature, making phone calls to voters, and lobbying federal agencies and members of Congress. According to the Center for Responsive Politics, total lobbying spending doubled from $1.65 billion to $3.27 billion between 2001 and 2011. It has thereby become difficult for voters to understand who is behind many political messages.[26]

Super PACs are the latest kind of political action committee on the scene. As independent expenditure-only committees, they can raise unlimited sums of money from corporations, unions, associations and individuals, then spend unlimited amounts to advocate or against political candidates. Super PACs are prohibited from donating money directly to political candidates, as traditional PACs can do. But they do have to report their donors to the Federal Election Commission on either a monthly or quarterly basis. As of January 26, 2012, there were 296 groups organized as Super PACs, with total expenditure of more than $40 million in the 2012 election cycle. Nine of the top Super PACs are conservative, only one liberal. Nor surprisingly, the top six Super PACs in terms of spending are all on the right and have very patriotic-sounding names (e.g. Restore Our Future, Winning Our Future, Make Us Great Again, Endorse Liberty, Our Destiny PAC, and Red, White and Blue).[27]

But these kinds of political fund-raising are a thoroughly bipartisan venture. In the midst of the Republican presidential primary season, as Mitt Romney's donations from Bain Capital employees have come under attack, we learn from the Center for Responsive Politics that Democrats have taken in even more than Republicans during the last three election cycles ($1.2 million vs. $480,000, mostly from senior executives). Since the beginning of 2007, Romney has accepted more than $166,000 in contributions from Bain Capital, while President Obama has collected more than $80,000 since that time.[28]

7. *Freeload: avoid corporate taxation as much as possible.*

Corporations have been expert at avoiding their fair share of U.S. taxes for many years, typically defending themselves by saying that "we are where the jobs come from." They have many ways of avoiding or limiting their taxes, including the use of tax havens overseas, lobbying the government for special tax breaks, and "innovative" accounting practices. General Electric (G.E.) is a poster child for success in tax avoidance: with worldwide reported profits of $14.2 billion in 2010, including $5.1 billion from domestic operations, it paid *no* U.S. taxes and even claimed a tax benefit of $3.2 billion! Its large tax department includes former officials from the IRS, the Treasury and virtually all of the tax-writing committees in Congress.[29]

To put this in perspective, these are the average tax rates (including payroll and income taxes), for middle class taxpayers, according to the nonpartisan Tax Policy Center:

- 12 percent for those with incomes between $34,000 and $60,000 a year
- 18.2 percent for those earning from $103,000 to $163,000 a year.[30]

Ironies permeate this whole story. Ronald Reagan was G.E.'s public face from 1954 to 1962, hosting the Sunday evening General Electric Theater on TV. Jeff Immelt, as the current CEO of G.E., heads the Obama Administration's Council on Jobs and Competitiveness. At the same time, his company employs more people overseas than in this country (152,000 vs. 133,000), with many overseas jobs formerly filled by U.S. workers, and threatens to move more jobs to Mexico, China and elsewhere. Meanwhile, one irony is that the right is starting to show cracks in its armor in its defense of business—small business vs. big business. In their defense of small business, Tea Party groups are attacking big corporations for "crony capitalism" over their use of government instead of the marketplace to do business.[31] And as public reaction against corporations avoiding taxes and parking their money offshore increases, corporations are lobbying for tax breaks to bring their money home, such as a "repatriation holiday" with a one-year tax of only 5.2 percent![32]

8. *Rig justice: make use of a conservative U.S. Supreme Court.*

Over the last 30 years, appointments to the highest court in the land have tended to be more conservative. The right has been quick to exploit its new opportunities, and a number of very conservative 5-4 rulings have resulted. Here are several examples:

- In its *Citizens United v. Federal Election Commission* ruling in 2010, the Supreme Court struck down 60 years of legal precedent prohibiting corporations from making campaign contributions in support of, or attacking political candidates. That 5-4 ruling reinforced the concept that corporations should have the rights of "persons" and can give unlimited amounts of money to political candidates of their choice.[33]
- In a 5-4 decision in 2011, the Supreme Court threw out a large employment discrimination class-action suit on behalf of up to 1.5 million female employees of Wal-Mart as it tightened the definition of what could qualify for a class-action suit. A more recent decision (*AT&T Mobility v. Conception*) ruled that corporations can use fine print in their contracts to deny people the right to band together for a class action lawsuit.[34]
- The drug industry profited from two other 2011 Supreme Court rulings, one limiting suits from people injured by their use of generic drugs, the other striking down a law banning some commercial uses of prescription drug data. In an effort to restrict drug companies from identifying what drugs physicians prescribe as part of their "detailing" and marketing to physicians, Vermont had passed such a law in 2007 that forbade the sale of prescription data by pharmacies and their use for marketing purposes. Thanks to the Supreme Court, that practice is now full speed ahead.[35]

As is the case with most other areas involving business interests and government, conflicts of interest with the judicial branch are also a problem, and often not addressed. Arguably, Clarence Thomas, the most conservative Justice on the Supreme Court, is a case in point. His conflicts of interest with his wife's increasing role in conservative politics have drawn scrutiny. His wife, Ginny Thomas, also an attorney, has been a leading advocate of the Tea Party since its inception. She has also been an outspoken opponent of the 2010 Patient Protection and Affordable Care Act (ACA), calling for its repeal as the Supreme Court plans to consider it in coming weeks. The fate of this bill, so-called "ObamaCare", will be a key issue in the 2012 elections. The appearance of conflict of interest has led 74 members of the House of Representatives to call on Clarence Thomas to recuse himself from voting on this issue. So far, there has been no reaction.[36]

At this writing, the Supreme Court is just weeks away from hearing a historic challenge to the ACA, particularly around the constitutionality of the individual mandate. A January 2012 Health Tracking Poll by the Kaiser Family Foundation found that nearly six in ten Americans expect the justices to base their decisions more on their personal ideology than on legal analysis; just 28 percent of respondents believed that the justices would make their decisions on the mandate without regard to politics and ideology.[37]

The above eight strategies used by the right over these last years, of course, do not tell the whole story. There are other areas that further their purposes. As the 2012 elections approach, one such example is the GOP's intensive effort to curtail voting rights around the country. The U.S. already has a poor record in voter turnout in presidential elections—never higher than 60 percent since 1968, much lower than participation levels in other Western democracies. The above-discussed ALEC is leading an effort to reduce turnout still further, particularly among the more disadvantaged in our society—the young, elderly and the poor. As ALEC's co-founder Paul Weyrich admitted three decades ago: "I don't want everybody to vote.... As a matter of fact, our leverage in the elections quite candidly goes up as the voting populace goes down." Under the pretense of preventing voter fraud, the right is now pushing various restrictive laws in many states that will limit voter turnout still further, such as by requiring certain kinds of voter ID, eliminating same-day voter registration, and cutting back on early voting. As one example, Texas has enacted a law that gives voters a ballot that qualifies voters if they have a military ID or a concealed-gun license while a college-ID will not![38]

WHERE DOES THIS LEAVE US NOW?

The class war that has been simmering over the last 30 years in this country is out in the open and is now readily obvious to most Americans. The right has made major gains to this point, even with the White House and Senate now in Democrats' control. Corporate interests have bought our government in both major political parties, and have taken us to this economic, social, and political crisis with both parties in ongoing gridlock. Financial reforms of Wall Street have been largely ineffective, and Main Street has lost much of what it had in previous times.

This is in sharp contrast to the post-World War II years in America. In their excellent 2010 book *Winner-Take-All Politics: How Washington Made the Rich Richer—and Turned Its Back on the Middle Class,* Jacob S. Hacker and Paul Pierson, professors of political science at Yale University and the University of California Berkeley, respectively, describe the years between the mid-1940s and about 1980 as years of "middle-class democracy." They recount how the American Legion effectively organized a national grassroots movement culminating in passage by Congress of the GI Bill, and how a Republican president (Eisenhower) lent strong support to the labor movement and chose to expand Social Security in the face of fierce opposition from business groups and conservative Republicans.[39] They also make these two observations about the two periods, then and now:

"The thirty-year war [since 1980] represents the least pleasant phase of a recurrent pattern in American democracy. Eras of drift punctuated by periods of renewal are what you get when you combine a dynamic market economy, an increasingly complex and fast-moving society, and a political system prone to stasis and to the protection of entrenched interests."[40]

And further: [As a result of the 2008 elections]

"A Democrat was in the White House. Democrats had control of both houses of Congress. But the president was hesitant to push for major economic reforms that would strain his mandate. The economy was delicate, the national debt large, right-wing opposition to his agenda strong. He also had conservatives to contend with in his own party. In the end, the president did not retreat— the challenges were far too great for that—but he trimmed his sails and sought reforms that fell well short of his and his party's grand ambitions."[41]

In this heated 2012 election cycle in the wake of the *Citizens United* ruling by the U.S. Supreme Court, political campaigns with massive Super PAC their elections. Without offering serious or credible programs to fix our economic and social problems, the right's main agenda seems to be to regain the White House and increase its strength in Congress at all costs.

All this is not new news. Some have seen this coming for years. Here is how Joseph Stiglitz, author of *Free Fall: Free Markets and the Sinking of the Global Economy*, sees how this has come about:

"Just a few years ago, a powerful ideology—the belief in free and unfettered markets—brought the world to the brink of ruin. Even in its hey-day, from the early 1980s until 2007, American-style deregulated capitalism brought greater material well-being only to the very richest in the richest country in the world.
Indeed, over the course of this ideology's 30-year ascendance, most Americans saw their incomes decline or stagnate year after year.
... Moreover, output growth in the United States was not eco-nomically sustainable. With so much of U.S. national income going to so few, growth could continue only through consump-tion financed by a mounting pile of debt."[42]

Jim Hightower, author of *Swim Against the Current: Even a Dead Fish Can Go with the Flow*, had this to say in May 2011 about where we now are:

"Workers in this country have been dramatically increasing their productivity since the highly ballyhooed economic recovery be-gan about twenty months ago, generating billions of dollars in new wealth. Yet, wages have stayed stagnant. Practically none of the increased wealth from worker productivity gains has gone to the workers. Instead, 94 percent of the money has been siphoned off by the corporate powers for such things as fattening profits at a record pace and jacking up CEO pay to exorbitant levels. Also, nearly $2 trillion of the gains have simply been stashed in the corporate vaults, rather than using it for wage hikes or new job creation.

And even the little bit of job creation that is taking place is "bottom heavy." Forty percent of the jobs lost in the recent economic crash were higher-paying positions, but 49 percent of the new jobs are low-paying.

Making the richest people richer is not a recovery—it's a robbery."[43]

And Arianna Huffington puts it this way:

"So the deck is stacked. The fix is in. The cards are marked. And the economy is rigged as a carnival ring-toss game.

But it's even worse than that. Corporate America's takeover of our democracy runs deeper than the simple quid pro quo of a donor swaying a politician. It has captured our leaders' hearts and minds. It's one thing for moneyed interests to be able to buy influence. It's another for that industry's agenda to become conventional wisdom across party lines." [44]

Figure 1.1 shows what has happened to income growth over the last three decades, with stark comparisons between the top 0.1 and 1 percent vs. the bottom 90 percent. The ratio of average CEO compensation to that of typical workers grew from 35 to 1 in 1978 to 243 to 1 in 2010.[45]

In response to the excesses of the right over these last years, we are now seeing many kinds of counterattacks being mounted in many areas. These efforts illustrate a new wave of resistance to conservative economic policies:

- A public backlash is now gaining momentum in the form of Occupy Wall Street protests around the country, 99/1 percent, and other grassroots activist efforts that will likely coalesce into a broader social movement to which both major parties will have to respond.

- Efforts are being made in Congress to bring forward a bill to make *Citizens United* unconstitutional.
- A divestiture movement against for-profit health insurers is gaining momentum.
- A recall election for Wisconsin Governor Scott Walker is in progress.

FIGURE 1.1

Income Growth 1979-2007

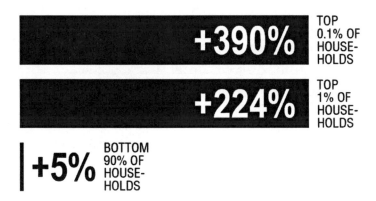

Source: Reprinted with permission from Ketcham, C. The new populists. *The American Prospect* 23 (1): 17, 2012.

Meanwhile, the blame game is in full force—an October 2011 *USA TODAY*/Gallup Poll found 78 percent of Americans blaming Wall Street for our economic problems, with 87 percent blaming the federal government.[46] Republicans blame Democrats, who in turn blame the Republicans. The electorate is increasingly polarized, with a major issue being the role of government in these challenging times.

How does all this affect health care in the fog of all-out class warfare? Health care reform, as with other of the nation's major problems, remains a hostage to the larger political landscape. As we will see in some detail in Chapter 11, the 2010 health care law was watered down and is not likely to make the kinds of reforms that are so urgently needed. Fundamental questions about health care reform have still not become part of the political debate, such as:

- Who is the health care system for—corporate interests or patients and families?
- Is health care a basic human need that should be available to all Americans based on medical necessity, not ability to pay?
- How can we expect the market to contain costs, when it hasn't done so over the last 30 years?
- Should we establish a health care system that provides universal access, is the most efficient, saves money, and gives optimal value and quality within available resources? Is so, in what ways?
- Should we perpetuate multi-payer financing with a failing private health insurance industry or switch to a more efficient, less expensive and more equitable single-payer financing system coupled with a private delivery system?

We will try to answer these questions in this book. And we will review in Chapter 12 some hopeful signs that suggest that the climate for progressive health care reform may be improving.

Our challenge, as an enlightened electorate in the midst of an important election season, is to separate claims and rhetoric from track record and facts. With that we move to the next chapter, where we will examine and rebut some of the major themes of the conservative mantra about markets and health care.

References

1. President Teddy Roosevelt, as quoted by Graves, L. About ALEC exposed. July 13, 2011. www.prwatch.org/node/10883
2. Giroux, HA. Surviving the second Gilded Age. *Truthout*, December 13, 2011.
3. Moore, M. Thirty years ago today: The middle class died. *Truthout*. August, 6, 2011
4. Wedel, JR. *Shadow Elite: How the World's New Power Brokers Undermine Democracy, Government, and the Free Market*. New York. Basic Books, 2009, pp 73-4.
5. Wysocki, B, Jr. Is U.S. Government 'Outsourcing its Brain'? *Wall Street Journal*, March 30, 2007:A1)
6. Booz Allen Hamilton. *The Globalization of White-Collar Work: The Facts and Fallout of Next-Generation Offshoring*. 2006. www.booz.com

7. Hanna, J. *How Many U.S. Jobs Are 'Offshorable'?* Harvard Business School, December 1, 2008. www.hbswk.hbs.edu

8. Huffington, A. *Third World America: How Our Politicians Are Abandoning the Middle Class and Betraying the American Dream.* New York. Crown Publishers, 2010: p. 28.

9. Early, S. *The Civil Wars in U.S. Labor: Birth of a New Workers' Movement or Death Throes of the Old?* Chicago. Haymarket Books, 2011: p.32.

10. Weisman, R. Website exposes Chamber's 'snake oil' regulatory tour. *Public Citizen News* 31 (4): 24, July/August 2011.

11. Ibid # 4, pp 10-11.

12. Kelman, S. The IG ideology. *Washington Post*, April 4, 2007:A13.

13. Project on Government Oversight. Gutting Government Oversight: The Steve Kelman Ideology. POGO website, April 30, 200.

14. Krugman, P. Letting bankers walk. Op-Ed. *New York Times*, July 18, 2011: A17.

15. Galbraith, JK. In Moyers, B. *Bill Moyer's Journal: The Conversation Continues.* New York. The New Press, 2011, p 237.

16. Murphy, K. Single-payer & interlocking directorates. *Extra!,* August 2009, p. 7.

17. Alterman, E. How Rupert buys friends and influences people. *The Nation* 293 (9-10): 10, 2011.

18. Cutrone, C, Rendall, S. Deficit-obsessed media misinform on causes. *Extra!* 24 (9): 4, 2011.

19. Light, PC. *A Government Ill Executed: The Decline of the Federal Service and How to Reverse It.* Cambridge, MA. Harvard University Press, 2008.

20. Kosar, KR. *The Quasi Government: Hybrid Organizations with Both Government and Private Sector Legal Characteristics.* CRS Report for Congress. Washington, D.C. Congressional Research Service, updated January 31, 2008, Summary.

21. Ibid # 4, p. 77.

22. Ferguson, T. Posted prices and the Capital Hill stalemate machine. *The Washington Spectator* 37 (18): 1, 2011.

23. Pocan, M. Inside the ALEC dating service: How corporations hook up with your state legislators. *The Progressive* 75 (10): 19-21, 2011.

24. Wilce, R. ALEC corporations spend big in Washington. September 13, 2011. www.prwatch.org/node/11022

25. Manes, B. Hiding the sausage: How a well-funded right-wing organization is grinding out state laws. September 16, 2011. www.prwatch.org/node/11030

26. Center for Responsive Politics. Washington, D.C. Outside spending (http://opensecrets.org/outside spending/, accessed January 26, 2012.

27. Center for Responsive Politics. Super PACs.http://www.opensecrets.org/pacs/superpacs.php?cycle=2012.

28. Bolton, A. Bain gives more campaign money to Democrats than it does to Republicans. *The Hill*, January 19, 2012.

29. Kocieniewsky, D. G.E.'s strategies let it avoid taxes altogether. *New York Times*, March 24, 2011. www.nytimes.com/2011/03/25/business/economy/25tax.html

30. Saunders, L, Hughes, S. Buffett builds his tax-the-rich case. *Wall Street Journal*, October 13, 2011: B1.
31. Linebaugh, K. Tea-party attacks put G.E. on defense. *Wall Street Journal*, October 10, 2011: A1)
32. Kocieniewsky, D. Companies push for a tax break on foreign cash. *New York Times*, June 20, 2011: A1.
33. Weisman, R. Corporate focus. Shed a tear for democracy. *The Progressive Populist* 16 (3): 13, February 15, 2010.
34. Public Citizen, October 12, 2011. htpp://action.citizen.org/p/dia/action/public/?action_KEY=4150)
35. Liptak, A. Drug makers win two Supreme Court decisions. *New York Times*, June 24, 2011: B1.
36. Toobin J. Partners: Will Clarence and Virginia Thomas succeed in killing Obama's health-care plan? *The New Yorker*, August 29, 2011: 40-51.
37. Carey, M.A. Majority of Americans think ideology will affect High Court's ruling on health law. *Kaiser Health News*, January 26, 2012.
38. Caldwell, P. Who stole the election? Dominating many state legislatures, Republicans have launched a full-on assault on voting rights. *The American Prospect*, November, 2011: 8-13.
39. Hacker, JS, Pierson, P. *Winner Take All Politics: How Washington Made the Rich Richer—And Turned Its Back on The Middle Class*. New York. Simon & Schuster, 2010, p. 138-40.
40. Ibid # 39, p. 297.
41. Ibid # 39, p. 137.
42. Stiglitz, JE. The ideological crisis of Western capitalism. July 6, 2011.
43. Hightower, J. The waiting game. *The Progressive* 75 (5): 46, 2011.
44. Ibid # 8, p. 51
45. Ketcham, C. The new populists. *The American Prospect* 23 (1): 17, 2012.
46. Hampson, R. For fiscal mess, more blame Washington over Wall Street. *USA Today*, October 18, 2011: 1A.

CHAPTER 2

The Conservative Mantra—With Rebuttals

"Government is not a trade which any man or body of men has a right to set up and exercise for his own emolument, but is altogether a trust, in right of those by whom that trust is delegated, and by whom it is always resumeable. It has itself no rights; they are altogether duties."[1]

—Thomas Paine

"There are powerful forces, which have no commitment to the open society, ready to seize the moment to snuff out the last vestiges of democratic egalitarianism. Our bankrupt liberalism, which naively believes Barack Obama is the antidote to our permanent war economy and Wall Street fraud, will either rise from its coma or be rolled over by an organized corporate elite and their right-wing lapdogs."[2]

—Chris Hedges, fellow at the Nation Institute
and author of *Death of the Liberal Class, Empire
of Illusion,* and *The World As It Is: Dispatches
on the Myth of Human Progress*

These two comments illustrate the enormous gap between the kind of government we hoped for at the birth of our country and what we have today more than two centuries later. As we saw in the last chapter, we have already lost much of our supposed democracy to corporate governance as our political powers have been bought off to do its will.

Before we can have much success in countering the many bad effects of the disconnect between Wall Street and Main Street over health care or other parts of our society, we first need to examine the conservative mantra and subject it to scrutiny. This chapter identifies some of the major assertions of the right, with brief rebuttals based on track record and evidence.

THE CONSERVATIVE MANTRA

Some Overarching Themes

1. *The private marketplace is better than public programs—it is more efficient, offers more choice and value, is less bureaucratic— and is the American way!*

   In maintaining this drumbeat rhetoric about the superiority of the private marketplace to get things done better than by government, conservatives also suggest that this approach will save money.

   But whether we look at government contracts, private health insurance, the private Medicare prescription drug benefit, or any number of other examples, the cost is invariably higher with less accountability compared to publicly financed and completed projects. The U.S. government overpaid the private sector for federal projects by at least $26 billion in 2010[3], with the average contracted project costing 83 percent more than an equivalent government-run project.[4] That pattern even extends to private contracts for prison management. We are now learning that contracted prison management costs more to operate than state-run prisons, even though they cut costs by avoiding the sickest, most costly inmates.[5]

   Why this lack of savings when costs are cut? The very structure of business, especially those that are investor-owned, dictates this outcome, by requiring that profits be gained from the work, including from recouping padded administrative, marketing and other costs along the way.

   A good example of this is to compare traditional government-run Medicare against private Medicare programs. The public version is administered with an overhead costs no more than 3 percent and with a fairly comprehensive set of benefits. By comparison, private Medicare programs have demonstrated less efficiency, higher costs, and less value over the last three decades. A 2000 report by the Government Accounting Office found that one way in which privatized Medicare programs increase their profits is by avoiding sicker enrollees.[6] A 2011 study by the American Medical Association, found that commercial health insurers have a claims-processing error rate of 19.3 percent, adding about $1.5 billion in unnecessary administrative costs to the health care system.[7]

Turning to privatization more generally, a recent study by the Project on Government Oversight, a non-profit Washington, D.C. group, found that in 33 of 35 occupations studied, the government paid billions of dollars more to private contractors than it would have by doing the work itself. Market rhetoric holds that government workers are paid too highly, but the reality is the opposite— contractors charged the government more than twice the amount paid to federal workers.[8]

2. We need to have the smallest government possible.

This goal is absurd, disingenuous, and cynical on its face when we find, as we did in the last chapter, that conservatives and their corporate allies have succeeded in attracting up to three-fourths of the work of the federal government through outsourced contracts to the private sector.[9] Essentially, the right wants to "starve the beast" of government while exploiting taxpayers' money to the fullest, all the while denying who is paying for and doing the work.

3. Regulation impedes progress; deregulation spurs innovation.

We have heard this for years from corporate sources and their propaganda machine.

As the current election cycle gathers steam and in hopes of gaining traction in a time of high unemployment, the U.S. Chamber of Commerce has undertaken an unprecedented anti-regulation campaign portraying regulation as a job-killer. All this in blatant denial of the large role of poor government oversight of Wall Street that threw 8 million Americans out of work, or other regulatory lapses in recent years, such as the BP blowout and the Massey coal mine explosion.[10] Moreover, corporate America is sitting on its cash and continues to outsource jobs, while small business creates new jobs more effectively than corporations.

The argument that regulation restricts innovation can also be readily countered. Considering new drugs, for example, six out of every seven "new" drugs are no better than the older ones and may be riskier because of premature approval without an adequate safety experience. Many drug breakthroughs are developed overseas, and we have a comparatively permissive regulatory approval process. Serious drug reactions are the fourth leading cause of deaths in hospitals, right behind heart disease, cancer and stroke.[11]

4. *Entitlement programs are for freeloaders.*

This insinuation is both inaccurate and denigrative of beneficiaries of public programs to which they have contributed over the years. It is also unfair and unjust, as shown by Figure 2.1. Social Security and Medicare are no more "entitlements" than a 401(k) plan is. All three are funded by taxes or contributions that come out of working peoples' pockets. Just as a working person deserves a pension, so he or she deserves Social Security and Medicare.

FIGURE 2.1

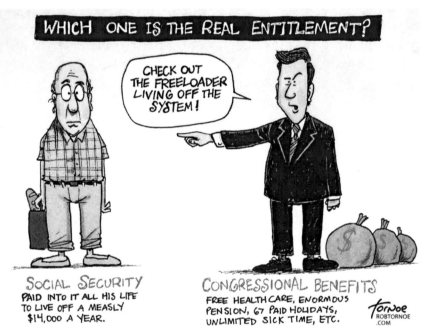

Source: Reprinted with permission from Rob Tornoe

Taking Social Security as an example, we can see that this claim is groundless and that former GOP presidential candidate Governor Rick Perry's ridicule of it as a Ponzi scheme was ill founded. Ellen Brown, news analyst at *Truthout*, reminds us that workers have paid into Social Security all their working lives and that it is not welfare but a debt due and payable. Congress passed it in 1935 as a retirement savings program.[12] A 2011 study by the Urban Institute concluded that the average worker retiring today will receive about the same amount he or she has paid in over the years, plus a 2 percent real interest rate (after inflation).[13]

5. Private investment and corporate profits drive the economy.

This is all we've told for the last 30 years—the *"trickle down"* theory of economics—a theory entirely discredited by experience. Between 1900 and 2000, real GDP per capita grew by more than 600 percent, while net business investment declined by 70 percent as a share of GDP. It is true that the private sector drove the economy in 1900, but most investment in 2000 was either from government spending from tax revenues or consumer spending. As an economic historian, James Livingston, professor of history at Rutgers University, gives us this historical perspective:

> "Corporate profits do not drive economic growth—they're just restless sums of surplus capital, ready to flood speculative markets at home and abroad. In the 1920s, they inflated the stock market bubble, and then caused the Great Crash.
>
> Since the Reagan revolution, these superfluous profits have fed corporate mergers and takeovers, driven the dot-com craze, financed the "shadow banking" system of hedge funds and securitized investment vehicles, fueled monetary meltdowns in every hemisphere and inflated the housing bubble."[14]

The 99 percent movement is no longer fooled by "trickle down" talk. In this Second Gilded Age, the gap between the 1 percent and the rest of us has never been wider, and it is now obvious that this gap is pulling us apart as a society. Without major reform, the American Dream is no longer possible for much of the population.

6. Corporations are people.

The notion that corporations should have the rights of natural persons, that they are persons, may seem outlandish. But it has been assumed by the U.S. Supreme Court for 125 years. In a 1886 case *Santa Clara County v. Southern Pacific Railroad*, the Supreme Court recognized (without debate) that corporations are persons for the purposes of the Fourteenth Amendment. Bancroft Davis, court reporter, summarized the case with a head nod to the Court's opinion that assumed that corporations are entitled to protection under the Fourteenth Amendment.[15] In later years, the Supreme Court has reiterated the concept that corporations are protected in many ways under the equal protection clause of the Constitution.[16]

The absurdness of corporations as persons was highlighted by GOP candidate former Massachusetts Governor Mitt Romney's recent video clip at the Iowa State Fair, in answer to a heckler:

> "Corporations are people, my friend... of course they are. Everything corporations earn ultimately goes to the people. Where do you think it goes? Whose pockets? People's pockets. Human beings, my friends." [17]

But as Richard Eskow of Campaign for America's Future points out:

> "Here's the paradox in this whole concept of "corporate personhood." When it comes to rights, Republicans say corporations are people. But when it comes to the responsibilities of personhood – like paying taxes, being sued for negligence or criminal manslaughter, that sort of thing – their response is 'Are you crazy? We're talking about *corporations* here, not people.'" [18]

Some Elements of the Mantra Related to Health Care

1. The competitive market will provide better value at less cost.

This has been repeated so many times over so many years by conservative market theorists as to amaze how this belief can be trotted out time after time. For the evidence is all to the contrary. We have had a deregulated "competitive" system for at least three decades, and what do we have to show for it but skyrocketing costs of health care, widespread disparities, unconscionable waste, and mediocre quality, despite our spending far more than any other nation in the world for health care.

Managed care of the 1990s promised us cost containment, which failed. Now we have "managed competition" and costs show no sign of being reined in. As Yogi Berra has said, "this is deja vu all over again." And we are reminded of the definition of insanity as doing the same things over and over again while expecting different results.

Beyond the failed track record of "market competition" over the last 30 years, here are several more specific rebuttals to this discredited theory:

- The free market allows, even encourages continuous escalation of prices by drug and medical device manufacturers, hospitals, other facilities, physicians and other members of the medical-industrial complex.[19]
- A nine-year study by the Community Tracking Study of 12 major U.S. health care markets has documented insufficient competition in each of these markets as a major barrier to efficiency and quality of care.[20]
- Consolidation among providers restricts choice and competition in many markets.[21]

2. Cost-sharing through "skin in the game" is an effective way to control health care costs.

This is the fundamental strategy in consumer directed health care as promoted by conservatives for years. It sees patients' choices to get care as a main reason for health care inflation through their "imprudent" choices. In their view, this is a moral hazard because people have no incentives to use health care sparingly, which results in over-utilizing services and expensive waste. Conservatives envision a world in which "empowered patients" shop for value in health care markets where prices are somehow transparent. But markets don't work that way for many reasons—sick patients are limited by the acuteness of their illness and availability of providers in their community, and information about costs and quality is hardly transparent. Moreover, we need to remind ourselves that *physicians,* practicing in a largely for-profit system with fee-for-service (FFS) reimbursement where the business model sets the bottom line, order and are responsible for most services that patients receive.

As a cost containment tool, cost-sharing doesn't work. Instead, it leads a growing number of patients to delay or forgo necessary care, resulting in later diagnosis of illness, higher costs down the road, decreased quality and worse outcomes of care.[22] In short, people die, often unnecessarily, from the way our system works. Cost-shifting just shifts more costs to patients and their families at a time when health care costs are the leading cause of personal bankruptcies, even among those with health insurance. A 2010 study of cost-sharing concluded that it is not necessarily an effective way to reduce health care spending, is not well-targeted to low-value services, and fails to distinguish between essential and non-essential services.[23]

3. First dollar insurance (without cost-sharing) coverage would break the bank.

This fear follows from the moral hazard argument that assumes that patients are the big culprits responsible for soaring health care costs. It is also tied to the right's fear of single-payer national health insurance, which would abandon cost-sharing altogether, as many other advanced industrial nations have done.

Here are three of the more obvious rebuttals to the fear that we can't afford to cover everyone without cost-sharing:

- When Canada introduced its single-payer system in the 1970s, there was a minimal increase in health care costs, hardly a rush to care, and most of that care was necessary; since then Canadians have had universal access to care with first dollar coverage and better outcomes of care while spending little more than one-half of what we spend on health care.[24]
- When Taiwan established its single-payer system in 1995, administrative costs were held at 2.3 percent, cost savings offset the incremental costs of covering all of the previously uninsured (again without cost-sharing), while access and outcomes of care improved dramatically.[25]
- We pay almost double what most other advanced nations, with less cost-sharing than we impose, spend each year for health care; despite our higher spending, we get less access and value for our money.

4. Everyone gets care anyhow.

Conservatives assume, since we have such a great health care system, that nobody goes without care. All they need to do is go to the E.R. or to one of our safety net facilities. This is patently untrue, as this one patient vignette (a representative one among many thousands) illustrates:

> *Kyle Willis, a 24-year old man from Ohio and a single father without health insurance, saw a dentist with a tooth ache who recommended removal of the tooth. Kyle could not afford that, so he waited. Later, after developing severe headaches and facial swelling, he went to an E.R., where antibiotics and pain medication were prescribed. But he could only afford one of the two, so he filled the pain prescription. But while the pain was relieved, the infection spread to his brain. He died, leaving a 6-year old daughter.[26]*

Similar stories are repeated every day in this country by the hundreds. If you go to the E.R., you can get very expensive, one-time care of acute problems, often without follow-up. If you are uninsured or on Medicaid, efforts to arrange follow-up are often fruitless, since many physicians will not see such patients. And drug prescriptions, as this example shows, are often unaffordable, so that patients have to make choices that may kill them.

So if you think that there is always a safety net available for you, think again, and just ask Kyle's family and the families of the 50,000 Americans who die each year without health insurance what they think. Meanwhile, as the shortage of primary care physicians becomes ever more critical and as emergency rooms close all over the country, the situation gets worse rather than better. In fact, the number of hospital emergency rooms in the U.S. dropped by 27 percent between 1990 and 2007. In fact, the hospitals that are most likely to close their E.R.s are for-profit hospitals and safety net hospitals in counties with a high poverty rate.[27] Moreover, with the increasing shortage of primary care physicians, E.R.s and urgent care centers are having increasing difficulty in arranging *any* follow-up care for their sick patients.

There is little security today for lower-income Americans, including a growing number of those in the middle class, when it comes to gaining necessary health care in our system based as it is on ability to pay, not medical need. We see every day that working hard, saving money and buying insurance is often not enough.

5. *The U.S. has the best health care system in the world.*

This belief among conservatives and market stakeholders persists without any consideration of the facts. The assumption is made that since we use so much technology in health care, have so many specialists and specialized facilities, and spend so much money, we must be the best in the world. That view is enhanced when some affluent visitors of other countries come here for their care. It is also enhanced by a blind belief in American "exceptionalism," as if we're naturally the best because that's the American way.

There is no question but that we are very good, and even best, at some things in our health care system. But to hold that we are categorically the best without defining what we mean by "best" is a big mistake. Those who think that we have the best health care in the world have to grapple with these questions:

- Why do we have the worst record for preventable deaths among 16 high-income countries? As reported by a 2011 study, deaths that are preventable by timely and effective care—mortality amenable to health care—is the worst in the U.S. among 16 high-income countries (95.5 deaths per 100,000 people), and the U.S. had the least improvement from 1997 to 2007 compared to those countries?[28]
- Why is it that up to one-third of all health care services in this country are either inappropriate or unnecessary, and some of them are actually harmful?[29]
- Why are we so bad at longevity compared to many other countries? It isn't because we are frugal—we spend about twice as much for health care as do other countries with much better longevity. (Figure 2.2)
- How is it that, comparing deaths among U.S. children younger than 5 to that of other countries, we rank 42nd? Our "best" system in the world puts us behind all of Western Europe and many other countries.[30]
- Why, among industrialized countries, do we have one of the highest mortality rates for dialysis patients?[31] And why is it that, in our great private system, the mortality rates in the two largest for-profit dialysis chains are 19 to 24 percent higher than not-for-profit chains?[32]
- While it is true that we have more specialists than other countries, why is it that the more specialists and the higher costs of care in an area, the lower is the quality of care?[33]
- Why do we let 50,000 Americans die each year (136 every day) for lack of health insurance?[34]

It is worth noting that the above statistics are not just dry and abstract numbers. Unfortunately for many Americans, they represent their deaths, either from lack of access or as a result of harmful outcomes of U.S. health care.

FIGURE 2.2

Per Capita Health Care Spending* and Life Expectancy, Selected Countries, 2000

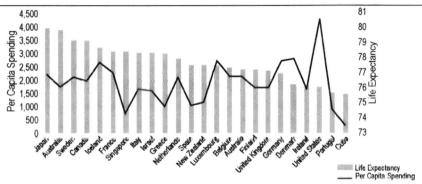

*Per Capita Spending is adjusted for Purchasing Power Parity (PPP) to eliminate the effect of short-term currency fluctuations.

Source: UC Atlas of Global Inequality, "Health Care Spending: Large Differences, Unequal Results." <ucatlas.ucsc.edu/spend.php> (November 15, 2007) Reprinted with permission.

6. *We can't have rationing of health care that would be imposed by a government-run system.*

This rhetoric draws from our mythical past (albeit briefly) picturing the rugged individualism of cowhands riding the western Plains, and lives on in our individualistic culture. It also draws from a libertarian view of a limited role of government, together with a certainty that the free market can best offer a menu of health care services from which patients, their families and caregivers are free to choose. It also supports the right of drug makers and other stakeholders on the supply side to bring to market whatever they like with minimal regulatory obstacles. All this ends up as an anti-government, anti-science mantra arguing against any independent science-based federal group making rationing decisions, and for a health care marketplace that denies care to the sick unless they can pay. Social Darwinism is here.

But obviously, rationing of one kind or another is necessary in any health care system. Resources to address the health care needs of any society are inevitably limited. The questions in rationing include who and how are decisions to be made, by what criteria, and how transparently? And further, how are the interests structured among those who make decisions—are they beholden to a government, or to investors? Most advanced countries provide universal access to a set of health care services of proven value, based on medical need. Here we refuse to recognize the disparities and inequities of our market-based system. If people can't afford essential care, that's their tough luck. Congress has not enacted legislation permitting an independent body to make coverage decisions based on efficacy and cost effectiveness.

Of course, any system of rationing is complex, involving economic, social, ethical and moral dimensions. If however we can agree that any system should be just and fair (i.e. American!), these words 24 years ago by Larry Churchill, well-known bioethicist at Vanderbilt University, still offer helpful guidance:

"A just health care system, whatever its final shape, requires a recognition of our sociality and mutual vulnerability to disease and death."[35]

WHERE NEXT: TOWARDS A COLLAPSE OF THE SYSTEM?

We can see that free market theories, despite insistence by the right over the last 30 years, do not work in health care. But that does not stop conservatives in this country, in an effort to expand their markets, from trying to export our failed policies overseas. A coalition of U.S. health care businesses, including the insurer UnitedHealth Group and the medical device maker Medtronic, are promoting the idea that they can add U.S. jobs in their sector by selling America's "health ecosystem" internationally. Working through the Alliance for Healthcare Competitiveness (AHC), they are proposing that the U.S. government build its foreign trade policy around the health care industry. All this under the banner of helping developing countries build "better" health care systems, while overlooking the problems that deregulated markets have produced here.[36]

Private health insurers are in a last-ditch battle to save themselves amidst soaring health care costs and dwindling prospects that either private of public payers can continue to purchase their underinsured, increasingly subsidized, products. They are already beholden to the federal government for continued subsidies and almost one half of their enrollees are in public programs, especially Medicare and Medicaid. The very expensive ObamaCare, as a handout to the insurance industry and other market stakeholders, will prove to be a large drain on federal and state coffers. Employers are continuing to cut their support of employer-sponsored health insurance. Other market stakeholders are starting to encounter less demand as more and more Americans can no longer afford health care.

No single factor will crash our health care system. But we may well be looking at a future where huge numbers of people cannot afford essential health care, and where the government can no longer afford its subsidies to the private sector. Combine that with a decreasing demand for health care services and we have a perfect storm brewing toward potential bursting of the health care bubble.

Strong and impressive as our medical-industrial-complex is, is that even a possibility? We already know that demand for health care is going down, mostly because of its increasing unaffordability. We can readily see the many signs that we are in a serious, ongoing recession, the worst downturn since the Great Depression, still without promising signs on the horizon. We know that our history is one of major changes and renewal in a different ways. And we know that almost all of the "experts" failed to predict the collapse of the housing bubble and our financial system in our recent past. So health care collapse is not just a scary and unfounded possibility.

We are surrounded by denial that markets have failed us, and that skyrocketing prices and costs of health care can go on forever. The right has no plan to fix our runaway system except by further privatizing public programs, including a voucher program for Medicare, and shifting an ever-increasing burden of health care costs to patients and their families. We should be heeding the words of Herbert Stein, an economist who served as chairman of the Council of Economic Advisors under Presidents Nixon and Ford, who tells us in what has been codified as Stein's Law:

"If something cannot go on forever, it will stop."[37]

As we look at the political discourse in this election season, one has to conclude that the right, disconnected as it is from reality, is still a dominant force in American politics. In its calls to prevent any future raise of the debt ceiling, making permanent all of the Bush tax cuts, and de-funding or repealing "ObamaCare," the Tea Party is moving Republicans farther right. As a result, fundamental health care reform is nowhere in the conversation. Paul Krugman sums up our political gridlock this way:

> "We have a crisis in which the right is making insane demands, while the president and Democrats in Congress are bending over backward to be accommodating—offering plans that are all spending cuts and no taxes, plans that are far to the right of public opinion."[38]

Figure 2.3 illustrates the present state of affairs.

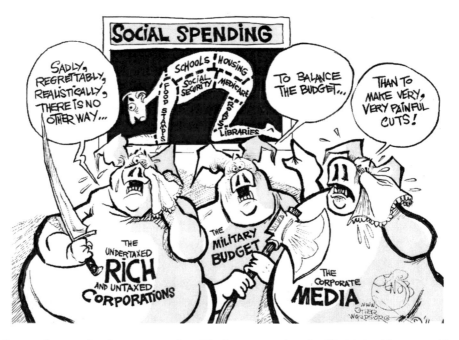

Source: *Reprinted with permission from The Progressive Populist* 17 (14), p. 15, August 15, 2011 and Khalil Bendib.

With this background, it is clear that we have a battle royal in progress between conservative forces on the right and liberal/progressive forces on the left. This is a work in progress, and the outcome is uncertain. Can there be a convergence of ideas between the right and left that will allow us to go forward? We will return to this question in Chapter 12.

For now, it is time to move to Part II, where we will examine in more detail just how market stakeholders serve themselves at our expense as they seek profits in a system where the time-honored not-for-profit service ethic of health care has disappeared into history.

References

1. Paine, T. *Collected Writings*. Foner, E. (Ed) New York. Literary Classics of the United States. Inc. 1995, p. 576.
2. Hedges, C. *The World As It Is: Dispatches on the Myth of Human Progress*. New York. Nation Books, 2011, p. 29.
3. Harper's Index. Harper's Research/U.S. Office of Management and Budget. *Harper's* 323 (1939): 86, 2011.
4. Harper's Index. Project on Government Oversight, Washington, D.C. *Harper's* 323 (1939): 86, 2011/
5. Oppel, RA, Jr. Private prisons found to offer little in savings. New York Times, May 19, 2011: A1.
6. General Accounting Office. *Medicare + Choice: Payments Exceed Costs of Fee-for-Service Benefits, Adding Billions to Spending*. GAO/HEHS-00-161. Washington, D.C.: Government Printing Office, 2000.
7. AMA. New AMA health insurer report card finds increasing inaccuracy in claims payment. June 20, 2011.
8. Nixon, R. Government pays more in contracts, study finds. *New York Times*, September 13, 2011: A 16.
9. Light, PC. *A Government Ill Executed: The Decline of the Federal Service and How to Reverse It*. Cambridge, MA. Harvard University Press, 2008.
10. Weissman, R. The GOP's deregulation obsession. *The Nation* 293 (18): 22, 2011.
11. Barry, P. The side effects of side effects. *AARP Bulletin* 52 (7): 14-6, 2011.
12. Brown, E. Forget compromise: the debt ceiling is unconstitutional. *Truthout*. August 1, 2011.
13. Urban Institute. Washington, D.C. htpp://www.urban.org/UploadedPDF/socialsecurity-medicare-benefits-over-lifetime.pdf
14. Livingston, J. It's consumer spending, stupid. *New York Times*, October 25, 2011.

15.	*Santa Clara County v. Southern Pacific Railroad*, 118 U.S. 394(http://supreme. justia.com/us/118/394/case.html) (1886)

16.	Corporate personhood. Wikipedia (htpp://en.wikipedia.org/wiki/Corporate_ personhood)

17.	Eskow, RJ. Shiny happy corporate people. *Truthout*, August 13, 2011.

18.	Ibid # 17.

19.	Weisbrot, M. Problems of U.S. health care are rooted in the private sector, despite right-wing claims. McClatchy-Tribune Information Services, July 20, 2011.

20.	Nichols, L et al. Are market forces strong enough to deliver efficient health care systems? Confidence is waning. *Health Aff (Millwood)* 23 (2): 8-21, 2004.

21.	Kronick, R, Goodman, DC, Weinberg, J, Wagner, E. The marketplace in health care reform. The demographic limitations of managed competition. *N Engl J Med* 328: 148, 1993.

22.	Geyman, JP. Moral hazard and consumer-driven health care: A fundamentally flawed concept. *Int. J Health Services* 37 (2): 333-51, 2007.

23.	Goodell, S, Swartz. L. Cost-sharing: effects on spending and outcomes. The Synthesis Project. Policy Brief No. 20, Robert Wood Johnson Foundation, December 2010.

24.	Armstrong, P, Armstrong, H, Fegan, C. *Universal Health Care: What the United States Can Learn from the Canadian Experience.* New York. The New Press, 1998, pp. 131-2.

25.	Lu, JR, Hsiao, WC. Does universal health insurance make health care unaffordable? Lessons from Taiwan. *Health Affairs* 22 (3): 77-88, 2003.

26.	Hubbard, L. Kyle Willis, Cincinnati man, dies from toothache, couldn't afford meds. *The Huffington Post*, September 3, 2011.

27.	Hsia, RC, Kellermann, AL, Shen, KY. Factors associated with closures of emergency departments in the United States. *JAMA* 305 (19): 1978-85, 2011.

28.	Nolte, E, McKee, M. Variations in amenable mortality—Trends in 16 high-income countries. New York. The Commonwealth Fund, September, 23, 20ll).

29.	Wennberg, JB, Fisher, ES, Skinner, Js. Geography and the debate over Medicare reform. *Health Affairs Web Exclusive* W-103, February 13, 2002.

30.	Rajaratnam, JK, Marcus, JR, Flaxman, AD, Wang, H, Levin-Rector, A et al. Neonatal, postnatal, childhood and under-5 mortality for 187 countries, 1970-2010: a systematic analysis of progress towards Millennium Development Goal 4.*The Lancet* 375: 1988-2008, 2010.

31.	Fields, R. In dialysis, life-saving care at great risk and cost *ProPublica*, November 9, 2010.

32.	Zhang, Y, Cotter, DJ, Thamer, M. The effect of dialysis claims on mortality among patients receiving dialysis. *Health Services Research* 46 (3): 747-67, 2011.

33.	Ibid # 29.

34.	Wolfe, SM. Outrage of the Month! 50 million uninsured equals 50,000+ avoidable deaths each year. *Health Letter* 28 (1): 11, January 12, 2012.

35.	Churchill, LR. *Rationing Health Care in America: Perceptions and Principles of Justice.* Notre Dame, KN: University of Notre Dame Press, 1987.

36. Kaiser Health News' Daily Report. Selling the American 'health ecosystem' internationally? September 27, 2011.

37. Stein, H. htpp://en.wikipedia.org/wiki/Herbert_Stein

38. Krugman, P. A cult of centrism, poisoning the American political system. Op-Ed, Krugman & Co. *Truthout*, August 2, 2011.

PART II

HOW HEALTH CARE MARKETS FAIL— AND CAN KILL YOU!

"[We have created] a society in which materialism dominates moral commitment, in which the rapid growth that we have achieved is not sustainable environmentally or socially, in which we do not act together as a community to address our common needs, partly because rugged individualism and market fundamentalism have eroded any sense of community and have led to rampant exploitation of unwary and unprotected individuals and to an increasing social divide. There has been an erosion of trust—and not just in our financial institutions. It is not too late to close these fissures."

—Joseph Stiglitz, Nobel laureate in economics and author of *Free Fall: America, Free Markets, and the Sinking of the World Economy* [1]

1. Stiglitz, JE. *Free Fall: America, Free Markets, and the Sinking of the World Economy*. New York. W. W. Norton & Company, Inc. 2010. 275-6.

CHAPTER 3

Profit-Driven Health Care Markets Drive Up Costs

"It's a popular idea: that Adam Smith's invisible hand would do a better job of designing care than leaders with [insurance] plans can. I do not agree. I find little evidence anywhere that market forces, bluntly used, that is, consumer choice among an array of products with competitors fighting it out, leads to the health care system you want and need. In the U.S. competition has become toxic: it is a major reason for our duplicative, supply-driven, fragmented care system...

Unfettered growth and pursuit of institutional self-interest has been the engine of low value for the U.S. health care system. It has made it unaffordable, and hasn't helped patients at all."

—Dr. Donald Berwick, former president and CEO of the Institute for Health Care Improvement and former Administrator of the Centers for Medicare and Medicaid Services (CMS) [1]

As inflation of health care costs continues unabated year after year, decade after decade in this country despite all efforts by policymakers and politicians to contain costs, health economists have struggled to understand why and to find a silver bullet.

All to no avail. Annual health care spending now totals $2.7 trillion, 17.7 percent of the nation's GDP, and $8,649 per capita. The Office of the Actuary of CMS projects that health care spending in the U.S. will reach 19.8 percent of GDP, $13,709 per capita by 2020. [2]

There are many factors that together account for our recalcitrant problem of health care inflation. For starters, they range across the incentives, behaviors and practices of physicians, other health care professionals, health care institutions such as hospitals and other facilities, industries within the medical-industrial complex, and patient behavior within social and cultural norms. How to make sense of all that? Which is most important? Actually, this is unknowable, for no studies have yet been able to tease out one factor more than others with any kind of precision. Most studies just consider one or a small number of factors in any given analysis.

In this and the following seven chapters in Part II of this book, we will describe various ways in which free markets in health care, contrary to classical market theory, do not contain costs through "competition." Instead we will find that they keep driving *up* costs, making them unaffordable for a growing part of our population, while decreasing patients' choice and quality of care.

We will not try to rank the relative importance of each factor directly, but these seven chapters together will add up to a picture that includes the most important ones. Our main task here is to lay out the dynamics that have resisted reform for so many years, so that we can develop an informed approach to reform in the last chapter.

This chapter has two goals: (1) to describe the five major trends that continue to drive health care costs upward and have resisted all previous efforts to contain their costs; and (2) to briefly summarize their impacts on access, affordability and quality of care that Americans receive.

MAJOR FORCES DRIVING UP HEALTH CARE COSTS

Most readers are fully aware of the steadily rising costs of health care, often in their own direct experience. But many will be less aware of the various forces driving health care inflation. Five leading dynamics are discussed here in an effort to show how widespread and relentless they are in foiling all past attempts to contain health care costs. From profit-driven insurance companies and other industries that make up the medical-industrial-complex to inventing new conditions for which treatments can be sold and conflicts of interest between physicians and industry, we will see how health care in this country soaks up an ever-larger part of our GDP and leaves many impoverished patients and families in its wake.

Let's take a look at each of these major dynamics in turn.

1. Profiteering by insurance companies.

Private health insurers in the U.S. over the last 40 years have been increasingly investor-owned and have become more and more expert at siphoning profits from health care transactions with enrollees of their policies to benefit their CEOs and shareholders. As is true for so many other areas of the medical-industrial-complex, their priorities are for maximal profits, highest returns to shareholders, and paying out the minimum amounts on actual health care. Their success in these goals are confirmed by these measures:

- The nation's five largest for-profit insurers netted $11.7 billion in profits in 2010, up by 51 percent since the start of the recession in 2008; Cigna's profits were up by 361 percent over 2008![3]
- Even with a marked falloff in enrollees' claims for health care during the recession, insurers kept on proposing double-digit premium increases.[4]
- CEOs of the country's five largest insurers took in $54.4 million in compensation in 2010, with Cigna's David Cordani leading the pack at $15.2 million.[5]

Insurers have a full quiver of strategies to limit their payments for health care while chasing profits. Standard ways include initial denial of coverage, denial of claims ("denial management" in the industry's jargon), adding new restrictions in fine print (such as steep co-payments for top-tier hospitals or drugs), and cancellation of policies. And the industry is adept at coming up with new and less recognized ways of enriching itself while claiming "service" to patients. Here is one example:

- A recent and growing trend is for insurers to create wholly-owned subsidiaries ("captive insurance companies"), which assume the risks of its parent company in exchange for a pre-determined premium payment. Captives are real insurance companies, and are really a form of self-insurance. They protect parent companies from risk and also allow insurers to avoid public oversight, since financial statements of captives remain confidential. Aetna recently used a subsidiary to re-finance a block of health insurance policies, thereby saving $150 million by not having to maintain conventional reserve requirements for those policies.[6]

As a result of its business practices over many years that limit access and restrict care for its own profit, the health insurance industry in this country is held in low public esteem—in a 2009 Harris poll, only 7 percent of 2,300 randomly selected respondents believed the industry to be honest and trustworthy.[7]

2. For-profit investor-owned industries.
The industries that collectively make up the medical-industrial complex are often for-profit, with an allegiance to shareholders over patients. In each case, they have developed their own clever techniques to milk more profits and "efficiency" from their delivery of services to patients. These are some of the ways that this is done in various industries:

- *Managed care organizations.* Whether health maintenance organizations (HMOs) or preferred provider organizations (PPOs), the majority that are investor-owned have a range of methods to increase their profits at the expense of patients, including padding their administrative costs, reducing their medical loss ratios (MLRs, the amounts spent on direct medical care), undertreatment and denial of services[8], and disenrollment of sick enrollees.[9]
- *Hospital chains and for-profit hospitals.* When hospital chains buy up a hospital, they make changes that illustrate their quest for profits above service to patients. As one example, when Hospital Corporation of America (HCA), the largest hospital chain in the country, took over Good Samaritan Health System in San Jose, California, nursing positions were cut, overnight housekeeping was eliminated, quality of care was compromised, and charity care was reduced. In another takeover of a Florida hospital, the emergency room was closed, requiring a 45-minute drive to the nearest emergency room during the resort town's busy season.[10]

For-profit hospitals can also increase their profits by purchasing other facilities, such as affiliated clinical laboratories, imaging centers, ambulatory surgery centers, rehabilitation, long-term care, and/or psychiatric facilities. Such control gives them new ways to build other revenue streams while expanding their market share. So-called specialty hospitals, most commonly for cardiac and orthopedic surgery care, allow physicians to "triple dip," padding their income by providing services as well as through their ownership and investor roles. By specializing in only a limited range of services, specialty hospitals are also able to avoid any obligation to maintain a money-losing emergency department.

- *Nursing homes.* About two-thirds of U.S. nursing homes are investor-owned, but because much of their business is dependent on Medicaid funding, this is an especially challenging market for them. A major strategy to cut costs and increase revenues is to cut back on nursing staff.
- *Dialysis centers.* About 85 percent of the nation's dialysis centers are investor-owned. Fresenius Medical Care North America is the dominant company, with more than 1,000 dialysis clinics. Compared with not-for-profit dialysis facilities, for-profits have been found to increase their profits by using shorter dialysis periods and reusing manufactured dialyzers that are labeled for single use in only one patient.[11] Another way to increase profits, exposed in a recent whistle-blower lawsuit, is to game a reimbursement policy by charging for unused portions of drug vials, with the size of the vials selected for maximal profits on unused drugs (e.g. using a 100 mg vial of Venofer, an iron drug, when only 25 mg was actually administered).[12]
- *Hospice.* The hospice movement, only 40 years old in the U.S., began as a largely volunteer-run, community-based, patient-centered movement in the tradition of the original concept pioneered by Dame Cicely Saunders, founder of St. Christopher's Hospice in a suburb of London in 1967. But, as with other parts of our health care system, this has all changed. An excellent recent article on the history and present status of hospice in this country traces the increasing commercialization of hospice. Its authors, Joshua Perry and Dr. Robert Stone, note that 52 per-

cent of hospices are now for-profit. Compared to not-for-profit hospices, their for-profit counterparts generate higher revenues in a number of ways—selectively recruiting the most profitable patients with the longest stays (e.g. favoring dementia patients over those with cancer), payment of lower salaries, and providing fewer benefits to less-skilled staff (fewer clinicians, registered nurses and medical social workers).[13] A 2004 report by the Government Accountability Office (GAO) is a measure of their success—between 1992 and 2002, the number of Medicare-participating hospices grew by almost 90 percent to 2,275. Medicare payments for hospice care increased by five-fold to about $4.5 billion; from 2001 to 2008, the hospice industry grew by 128 percent to more than 3,300 locations, with the for-profit sector accounting for almost all of that increase.[14,15]

- *Drug industry.* We have already noted some of the ways by which the drug industry has for many years led the field in terms of profitability. This is no accident, for the industry has many ways at its disposal to maximize its profits. Here is just a partial list of ways about which many of us may be unaware:
  - false and misleading advertising hyping benefits and downplaying risks[16]
  - delayed or inaccurate reporting of risks and adverse outcomes[17]
  - gaming the system to extend patents and monopolies beyond 17 years or blocking competitors from acquiring patents[18]
  - commissioning ghost writers to write articles promoting their products without regard to their risks[19]
  - publishing favorable research results while suppressing publication of negative results[20]
  - attempts to harass, intimidate or discredit investigators who conduct unfavorable studies[21]
  - manipulating the process of clinical practice guideline development for marketing purposes[22]
  - sharing non-public scientific date with selected Wall Street analysts while calling on them not to share the information[23]

- *Medical device industry.* The medical device industry operates in a large market with products ranging from cardiac pacemakers and implantable defibrillators to lasers, hip and knee replacements. About one-half of them are considered low-risk, while higher risk devices must undergo some level of review by the FDA. As with the drug industry, this review tends to be industry-friendly and often fails to be rigorous. A measure of the risks involved is suggested by the recall of more than 1,000 medical devices each year.[24]

As we've seen with drug companies, medical device manufacturers frequently try to extend their markets as long as possible even when their products have been found defective or harmful. They have various means at their disposal, including delaying notification of the FDA about negative experiences with their products, continued marketing beyond adverse reports, and seeking protection from willing legislators. Examples of such delaying actions in recent years include Pfizer's defective Bjork-Shiley heart valve [25] and Guidant's short-circuiting implantable heart defibrillators.[26]

3. Medicalization

This may surprise many as one of the main causes of health care inflation, since it has become so much a norm in today's culture. But it plays a large and under-recognized role in pushing health care costs endlessly up. By *medicalization* we mean the process by which non-medical problems become defined and treated as medical problems, usually in terms of disorders and illness. In this way, the boundaries of health care are expanded by many contributing factors, including advances in technology, professional and industry interests, market forces, advertising and educational campaigns, and favorable reimbursement policies by payers. More than 20 years ago, Arthur Barsky, a psychiatrist at Harvard Medical School, described the dynamics of medicalization in this way:

"Health is industrialized and commercialized in a fashion that enhances many people's dissatisfaction with their health. Advertisers, manufacturers, advocacy groups, and proprietary health care corporations promote the myth that good health can be purchased; they market products and services that purport to deliver the consumer into the promised land of wellness. A giant medical-industrial complex has arisen, composed initially of for-profit health care corporations such as free-standing ambulatory surgery centers, free-standing diagnostic laboratories, home health care services, and of course proprietary hospitals. But the market is so lucrative that the products of the medical-industrial complex now range all the way from do-it-yourself diagnostic kits to "lite" foods, from tooth polish to eye drops, from health magazines to Medic-Alert bracelets, from exercise machines to fat farms." [27]

Combine continuously widening boundaries of what we mean by "health care" (whether indicated by clinical evidence or not) with a deregulated supply-side, market-oriented system driven by an insatiable need for new revenue streams by selling a wider array of "products"— and you have the perfect prescription for uncontrollable health care costs stretching as far the eye can see.

As described in my 2002 book *Health Care in America: Can Our Ailing System Be Healed?* there are five major ways, sometimes overlapping, by which expansion of health care boundaries takes place: [28]

- *Medicalizing the culture.*
  At one end of life's spectrum, anesthesia for childbirth, as well as the big increase in Caesarian sections and infant bottle feeding give us examples of how obstetric practice and newborn care have changed greatly over the years. At the other end of the life cycle, most will agree that the process of dying has been medicalized way beyond earlier approaches to end-of-life care, most recently with some suggesting that grieving should become a treatable disorder.[29]
- *Applying new technology.*
  The introduction of continuous fetal monitoring of women in labor in the 1970s, though it did lead to improvements in the infant mortality rate, nevertheless converted about one-quarter of pregnancies to a surgical problem.
- *Refining diagnostic tools.*
  Here we struggle with the definition of "normal" as diagnostic procedures inevitably identify more disease, often before

it becomes symptomatic. Where does normal leave off and "disease" start? Examples of the problem include the discovery of a bulge in a lumbar disc in patients without back pain (one-half of young adults) and knee abnormalities in one-quarter of asymptomatic young adults. More sensitive diagnostic tests often lead to unnecessary and inappropriate follow-up and treatment of asymptomatic conditions.

- *Changing definitions of existing diseases.*
  What might seem as a modest definitional change can lead to big changes in medical practice and prevalence of a "disease." As examples, if we change the definition of high cholesterol from total cholesterol of more than 240 mg/dl to above 200 mg/dl, the prevalence of hypercholesterolemia goes up by 86 percent; changing the definition of overweight from a body mass index of more than 27 kg/m^2 to 25 kg/m^2 increases its prevalence by 42 percent.[30] In both instances, nothing has changed, but the scope of the problems are defined as being much bigger.

- *Defining new diseases.*
  Some examples of problems that can be questioned as actual disease include hypoglycemia, mild mitral valve prolapse, irritable colon and premenstrual syndrome. Somatic complaints are an especially difficult area to distinguish from disease, since they are very common, lead somatizing patients to frequent physician visits, and are usually not associated with disease. The drug industry is especially "innovative" in building new markets for their drugs through "disease awareness" programs and "disease branding." One example is the current promotion of low testosterone ("low T") as a disorder needing treatment in middle-age males. Another is the marketing campaign by Pharmacia promoting its drug Detrol for what physicians knew as *urge incontinence*. By re-branding (and de-stigmatizing) this common but embarrassing complaint as *overactive bladder—* Pharmacia "created" a new disease and a mass-market opportunity.[31]

4. Conflicts-of-interest between physicians and industry.

As described in my 2008 book *The Corrosion of Medicine: Can the Profession Reclaim Its Moral Legacy?*, a cozy relationship of mutual self-interest between many physicians and industry has become an entrenched norm in our market-based system. As we have seen, physicians are increasingly employed by one or another part of a bigger system oriented to maximizing of profits, whether by hospitals, hospital systems, HMOs, or other parts of the medical-industrial complex.

These examples show that conflicts-of-interest (COIs) are not just a matter of "a few bad apples," but are instead a common and intentional part of the money culture of medicine:

- Physicians who own their own CT and other imaging equipment order two to eight times more imaging tests as those who do not own such equipment, altogether amounting to some $40 billion worth of unnecessary imaging each year.[32]
- Physician-owned specialty hospitals for cardiac care lead to duplication of services without significant increased access. They also lead to increased rates of procedures, especially angioplasties and stents.[33,34]
- Overuse of anemia drugs for cancer patients continues despite warnings by the FDA of their adverse risks of stroke or heart attack. This pads the incomes of prescribing oncologists while wasting some $60 billion over the last 20 years.[35]
- There are now surgeon-owned implant companies for spinal surgery in 20 states, and they are spreading into other clinical areas, such as hip, knee and cardiac surgery. In this way, surgeons take a "double cut" by using devices made by their own companies.[36]
- Despite attempts in recent years to reduce or eliminate COIs among physicians serving on clinical practice guideline committees, they are still very common. This is illustrated by a 2011 report finding 8 of 19 panel members with such conflicts on an NIH obesity panel and 5 of 17 panel members on a hypertension panel; surprisingly, this included the chairpersons of both panels.[37]
- There are more than 4,200 ambulatory surgery centers (ASCs) across the country. These are typically privately owned between hospitals and physicians, sometimes owned entirely by physicians or investor-owned companies. The most successful ASCs have a profit margin of more than 20 percent. COIs are so pervasive that a 2003 article in *Medical Economics* gave advice

to physician investors on how to avoid being targeted by anti-kickback regulations aimed at curtailing kickbacks.[38]

- Phase IV drug trials have become a lucrative source of income for participating physicians. These are uncontrolled registry drug trials, with minimal rigor, funded by drug companies with the intent to build a large following among physicians and patients.[39]
- Large gifts and investments by industry in university academic health science centers under so-called institutional academic industry relationships (IAIRs) are another common source of often unrecognized COIs. A 2004 report of a comprehensive study of four unnamed centers revealed a variety of ways in which these conflicts among institutional leaders and researchers raise concerns over the integrity of their research.[40]
- Even the growing field of bioethics has become embroiled in controversy over COIs. Many companies and institutions have hired bioethicists, and some have even started their own for-profit consultation businesses. As a result of this transition, sociologist Jonathan Imber has called bioethics "the public relations division of modern medicine."[41] In his excellent book *White Coat Black Hat: Adventures on the Dark Side of Medicine,* Dr. Carl Elliott, professor at the University of Minnesota's Center for Bioethics, points out the obvious:

"An ethicist can bite the hand that feeds it for only so long before the food stops coming."[42]

5. Inappropriate and unnecessary care.

The fee for service (FFS) system of reimbursement of health care services creates many ways by which physicians and their employers can game the system in their own self-interest. These include providing more services than are necessary, increasing the frequency of visits, and exaggerating the number or complexity of problems dealt with during visits ("upcoding"). By contrast, physicians paid by salary have no such incentives to overcharge by billing for more services than are necessary.

These markers indicate the magnitude of this problem:

- Studies by a well-known research group at Dartmouth Medical School have shown that about one-third of all health care delivered in the U.S. appears to be either inappropriate or unnecessary.[43]

- That same health services research group estimates that about 40 percent of all specialist visits and 25 percent of hospitalizations are unnecessary.[44]

- A 2010 report of a national study of nearly 400,000 patients who underwent elective cardiac catheterization with no known history of coronary artery disease found that only about one-third actually had significant obstruction of their coronary arteries; in the 1990s, the figure for those who actually had obstruction of their coronary arteries was between 70 and 90 percent, this suggesting that invasive and potentially hazardous diagnostic cardiac workups are being overused.[45]

- Angioplasty and stent placement are also overdone; many cardiologists place stents if the coronary angiogram shows some narrowing, even in patients *without* symptoms, and many hospitals use consent procedures that permit such same-day procedures without enabling patients to have full informed consent of their therapeutic choices.[46]

- Many surgical procedures are carried out without evidence of their therapeutic benefit, as exemplified by popular hip impingement or bone-shaving surgery for hip problems[47] as well as extremely aggressive procedures involving extensive surgery and heated chemotherapy (Hipec) for some colorectal and ovarian cancers.[48]

- Dr. James Andrews, a highly respected sports medicine specialist, suspected that MRIs are being overused in shoulder problems of athletes. In testing out his suspicion, he found that asymptomatic pitchers without injuries or pain had abnormalities discovered by MRIs of shoulder cartilage in 90 percent and of rotator cuff tendons in 87 percent. As he observed: "If you want an excuse to operate on a pitcher's throwing shoulder, just get an MRI."[49]

FREE-WHEELING HEALTH CARE MARKETS
IS WHAT WE GET WORTH THE MONEY?

We can see from the above that much of the medical-industrial complex, particularly those parts that are investor-owned, serve themselves above the interests of patients and families. Of course, they deny this and conduct ongoing PR and disinformation campaigns as they posture themselves in the public interest.

As the various industries within the medical-industrial complex continue to do well, there is increasing evidence that this health care "bubble" may be headed for a the same kind of bust that hit the housing and financial markets. We have only to look at the behavior of patients for clues to this prospect. As the recession rolls on and deepens for many Americans, they delay or forgo health care at an increasing rate. They are less able to afford the out-of-pocket costs of care (and insurance), even when they are "insured."

In a country where wealth has increasingly transferred up to the rich, this recession hits most Americans hard. That is especially true with the current conditions, four years after this recession, where unemployment has been above 8 percent for the last four years (double that including those who have given up on getting a job), the first time this has happened since the Great Depression. In these times, it is no wonder that people are cutting back on everything, including health care expenditures. The ability of the medical-industrial-complex to continue its rapacious growth on the backs of the 99 percent seems dim at best.

As we will continue to point out throughout this book, as costs go up and become unaffordable, access to care drops off while quality and outcomes of care suffer. It is clear that the United States will continue to be at the bottom of the pack in cross-national comparisons of health care systems in developed countries, even though we spend about double what other industrialized countries spend on health care.

Across the board, we now have solid evidence that for-profit investor-owned parts of our market-based system provide *worse* quality of care. Because our system has a gargantuan private sector plus very large public sectors (especially Medicare, Medicaid, and the Veterans Administration), comparisons between for-profit chains and their not-for-profit counterparts tell the story:

- *HMOs*: Higher overhead (15 to 25 percent higher for some of the largest HMOs) with worse outcomes on 14 of 14 quality indicators reported to the National Committee for Quality Assurance [50]
- *Hospitals*: Costs 3 to 13 percent higher, with higher overhead, fewer nurses, and death rates 6 to 7 percent higher [51-53]; moreover, not-for-profit Veterans Health Administration (VHA) hospitals

have been shown to have better quality of care than hospitals in the private sector[54], while a 2011 study of the VHA system documented higher rates of curative resection for colon cancer, recommended chemotherapeutic regimens for hematologic neoplasms, and bisphosphonate use for multiple myeloma.[55]

- *Nursing homes*: in a 2002 study, lower nurse staffing levels and worse quality of care compared to their not-for-profit counterparts, with deficiencies even to the point of putting some patients at risk for serious injury or death;[56] a 2009 study found less nursing care, higher prevalence of pressure ulcers, more frequent use of physical restraints and more quality violations in government regulatory assessments in for-profit nursing homes.[57]
- *Dialysis centers*: death rates 30 percent higher, with 26 percent fewer referrals for transplants in a 2002 study.[58]
- *Hospices*: For-profits provide a full range of end-of-life services only half as often (e.g. palliative radiation therapy for cancer and family counseling).[59]

In view of these kinds of findings, Dr. Gordon Guyatt, professor of medicine at McMaster University in Hamilton, Canada, world leader in evidence-based medicine, and senior author of the 2009 study of nursing homes noted above, has this to say about for-profit health care:

"Our results should raise serious concerns about for-profit care, whether in nursing homes, hospitals, surgi-centers, or other out-patient facilities. It is time to base health care policy on evidence, not ideology." [60]

In the following chapters, we will examine other ways in which the supply side of health care delivery accentuates its profits over the needs and interests of patients on the receiving end. But wait a minute. Isn't market competition a great thing? In the next chapter we turn to find how much latitude supply-siders in the market have to set their own prices in our laissez faire "system."

References

1. Berwick, DM. A transatlantic review of the NHS at 60. *British Medical Journal* 337 (7663): 212-4, 2008.
2. Office of the Actuary, CMS. National health spending projections through 2020. *Health Affairs*, July 28, 2011.
3. Health Care for American Now! Health insurers pocketed huge profits in 2010 despite weak economy. March 3, 2011.
4. Abelson, R. Health insurers making record profits as many postpone care. *New York Times*, May 13, 2011.
5. Executive PayWatch, AFL-CIO, 2011.
6. Walsh, MW, Story, L. Seeking business, states loosen insurance rules. *New York Times*, May 8, 2011.
7. Wolfe, SM. Outrage! The health insurance industry. *Health Letter* 26 (9): 11, 2010.
8. Court, J, Smith, F. *Making a Killing: HMOs and the Threat to Your Health.* Monroe, ME. Common Courage Press, 1999.
9. Morgan, RO, Virnig, BA, DeVito, CA, Persily, NA. The Medicare HMO revolving door—the healthy go in and the sick go out. *N Engl J Med* 337: 169-75, 1997.
10. Ginsberg, C. The patient as profit center: Hospital Inc. comes to town. *The Nation*, November 18, 1996.
11. Himmelstein, DU, Woolhandler, S, Hellander, I. *Bleeding the Patient: The Consequences of Corporate Health Care.* Monroe, ME. Common Courage Press, 2001.
12. Pollack, A. Lawsuit says dialysis drugs were wasted to buoy profit. *New York Times*, July 27, 2011: B1.
13. Perry, JE, Stone, RC. In the business of dying: Questioning the commercialization of hospice. *Journal of Law, Medicine & Ethics*, Summer 2011: 224-34.
14. MedPAC. Report to the Congress: Medicare Payment Policy, Hospice, March 2010, p. 141.
15. von Gunten, CF. Profit or not-for-profit: who cares? *Journal of Palliative Medicine* 11 (7): 954, 2008.
16. Wolfe, SM (ed). Outrage of the month. The causes of mis-prescribing and over-prescribing. Washington, D.C.: *Health Letter.* Public Citizen's Health Research Group, May 2005: 9-10.
17. Wolfe, SM (ed) Sleight-of-hand. Merck contemplated Vioxx reformulation in 2000 while denying risk. Washington, D.C.: *Health Letter*, Public Citizen's Health Research Group, August 2005: 1-2.

18. Public Citizen Report, November 9, 2001,

19. Larkin, M. Whose article is it anyway? *Lancet* 353: 136, 1999.

20. Lexchin, J, Bero, LA, Djulbegovic, B, Clark, O. Pharmaceutical industry sponsorship and research outcome and quality: a systematic review. *British Medical Journal* 326: 1167, 2003.

21. Rennie, DM. Thyroid storm. *JAMA* 277: 1242, 1997.

22. Erichacker, PQ, Natanson, C, Danner, RL. Surviving sepsis—practice guidelines, marketing campaigns, and Eli Lilly. *N Engl J Med* 355 (16): 1640-2, 2006.

23. Abboud, L, Zuckerman, G. Drug maker draws heat for sharing non-public data with stock analysts. *Wall Street Journal*, October 4, 2005.

24. Feigal, DW, Gardner, SN, McClellan, J. Ensuring safe and effective medical devices. *N Engl J Med* 348: 191, 2003.

25. Palast, G. *The Best Democracy Money Can Buy.* Sterling VA: Pluto Press, 2002.

26. Burton, TM, Mathews, AW. Guidant sold heart device after flaws. *Wall Street Journal*, June 2, 2005: D3.

27. Barsky, AJ. The paradox of health. *N Engl J Med* 318:414-18, 1988.

28. Geyman, JP. *Health Care in America: Can Our Ailing System Be Healed?* Woburn, MA. Butterworth-Heinemann, 2002, pp.29-41.

29. Carey, B. Grief could join list of disorders. *New York Times*, January 24, 2012: A1.

30. Schwartz, LM, Woloshin, S. Changing disease definitions: Implications for disease prevalence. Analysis of the Third National Health and Nutrition Examination Survey. *Eff Clin Pract* 2 (2): 80, 1999.

31. Associated Press. FTC clears way for Pfizer acquisition of Pharmacia. *USA Today*, April 14, 2003.

32. Bach, PB. Paying doctors to ignore patients. *New York Times*, July 24, 2008.

33. Lucas, FL, Slewers, A, Goodman, DC, Wang, D, Wennberg, D. New cardiac surgery programs established from 1993 to 2004 led to little increased access, substantial duplication of services. *Health Affairs* 30 (8): 1569-74, 2011.

34. Nallamothu, BK, Rogers, MA, Chernew, ME, Krumholz, HM, Eagle, KA et al. Opening of specialty cardiac hospitals and use of coronary revascularization in Medicare beneficiaries. *JAMA* 297 (9): 962-8, 2007.

35. Harris, G. F.D.A. urges less use of anemia drugs. *New York Times*, June 25, 2011: B1.

36. Carreyrou, J, McGinty, T. Taking double cut, surgeons implant their own devices. *Wall Street Journal*, October 8, 2011: A1.

37. Wilson, D. Conflicts on guideline panels. *New York Times*, November 3, 2011: B1.

38. Luxenberg, S. Invest in a surgicenter? *Medical Economics*, December 5, 2003, pp. 60-65.

39. Borfitz, D. Can "phase IV" trials work for you? *Medical Economics*, June 6, 2003, pp. 58-67.

40. Campbell, EG, Weisman, JS, Clarridge, B, Yucal, R, Causino, N et al. Institutional academic industry relationship: Results of interviews with university leaders. *Accountability in Research* 11: 103-18, 2004.
41. Imber, J. Medical Publicity before Bioethics: Nineteenth-Century Illustrations of Twentieth-Century Dilemmas. In DeVries, R, Subedi, J (eds). *Bioethics and Society: Constructing the Ethical Enterprise.* New York. Prentice Hall, 1998: p. 30.
42. Elliott, C. *White Coat Black Hat: Adventures on the Dark Side of Medicine.* Boston. Beacon Press, 2010, p. 157.
43. Wennberg, JB, Fisher, ES, Skinner, JS. Geography and the debate over Medicare reform. *Health Affairs Web Exclusive* W-103, February 13, 2002.
44. Langreth, R. Useless medicine. *Forbes.* November 30, 2009, p. 66.
45. Patel, MR, Peterson, ED, Dai, MS, Brennan, JM, Redberg, RF. Low diagnostic yield of elective coronary angiography. *N Engl J Med* 362: 862-95, 2010.
46. Wolfe, SM. Many patients undergo unnecessary invasive cardiac procedures. *Health Letter* 27 (4):2-3, 2011.
47. Kolata, G. Hip procedure grows popular despite doubt. *New York Times,* November 16, 2011: A1.
48. Lerner, BH. The annals of extreme surgery. Op-Ed. New *York Times,* August 30, 2011: A21.
49. Kolata, G. Sports medicine said to overuse a popular scan. *New York Times,* October 29, 2011: A1.
50. Himmelstein, DU et al. Quality of care in investor-owned vs. not-for-profit HMOs. *JAMA* 282:159, 1999.
51. Silverman, EM et al. The association between for-profit hospital ownership and increased Medicare spending. *N Engl J Med* 341: 420, 1999.
52. Woolhandler, S, Himmelstein, DU. Costs of care and administration at for-profit and other hospitals in the United States. *N Engl J Med* 36: 769, 1997.
53. Yuan, Z. The association between hospital type and mortality and length of stay: a study of 16.9 million hospitalized Medicare beneficiaries. *Med Care* 38: 231, 2000.
54. Rosenthal, GE, Sarrazin, MV, Harper, DL, Fuehrer, SM. Mortality and length of stay in a veterans affairs hospital and private sector hospitals serving a common market. *J Gen Intern Med* 18: 601-8, 2003.
55. Keating, NL, Landrum, MB, Lamont, EB, Bozeman, SR, Krasnow, SH et al. Quality of care for older patients with cancer in the Veterans Health Administration versus the private sector: a cohort study. *Ann Intern Med* 54: 727-36, 2011.
56. Harrington, C, Woolhandler, S, Mullen, J, Carillo, H, Himmelstein, DU. Does investor-ownership of nursing homes compromise the quality of care? *Am J Public Health* 91: 1-5, 2001.
57. Comondore, VR, Devereaux, PJ, Zhou, Q, Stone, SB, Busse, JW et al. Quality of care in for-profit and not-for-profit nursing homes: systematic review and meta-analysis. *British Medical Journal* 339: 2732, 2009.

58. Devereaux, PJ, Schunemann, HI, Ravindran, M, Bhandari, M, Garg, AX et al. Comparison of mortality between private for-profit and private not-for-profit hemodialysis centers: A systematic review and meta-analysis *JAMA* 288: 2449, 2002.

59. Ibid # 12.

60. Guyatt, GH, as quoted in Science Daily. Nonprofit nursing homes provide better care, major study finds. August 19, 2009.

CHAPTER 4

The Price is Right (Unless You're the Patient): How Exploitive Pricing Works in a "Free Market" System

Of the many theories proposed for why health care spending continues to escalate at rates several times the cost of living, most have skirted the matter of prices themselves. But then a landmark article in *Health Affairs* in 2003 entitled *It's the Prices, Stupid: Why the United States is So Different from Other Countries*, brought the issue of pricing front and center. Based on a study of data from the Organization for Economic Cooperation and Development (OECD), Gerard Anderson, professor of health policy and management and international health at the Johns Hopkins University School of Public Health and Uwe Reinhardt, professor of economics and public affairs at Princeton University and colleagues compared health care spending patterns in 30 member countries in 2000. They also studied comparative health system capacity and use of medical services. Their findings were interesting:

- U.S. per capita spending is 44 percent higher than Switzerland (the next most expensive country), 83 percent higher than Canada, and 134 percent higher than the OECD median.
- Compared to Canada, the U.S. performs four times as many coronary angioplasties, twice the number of kidney dialyses, and has more than three times the number of MRI scanners per capita.

- Although by far the biggest spender, the U.S provides fewer services than the median OECD country—fewer physician visits per capita, fewer hospital admissions, and fewer hospital days per capita.
- Prices are more effectively controlled in Europe, Canada and Japan through more monopsonist market power on the buy side (i.e. one main purchaser—the government). The researchers concluded:

"Since spending is a product of both the goods and services used and their prices, this implies that much higher prices are paid in the United States than in other countries. But U.S. policymakers need to reflect on what Americans are getting for their greater health spending. They could conclude: It's the prices, stupid."[1]

We now have an important update in a new OECD report *Health at a Glance 2011: OECD Indicators*. Compared to five other OECD countries, we learn that U.S. spending on ambulatory care is almost 250 percent higher, hospital spending is more than 60 percent higher, and spending on pharmaceuticals and medical goods is also higher. All that in spite of the U.S. having less physicians per population, fewer physician visits and hospital beds, and shorter hospital stays. The report concluded that prices are an important cause of higher health care spending in this country.[2]

In this chapter we will (1) examine the extent to which four major parts of the medical-industrial complex—providers, hospitals, drug manufacturers and insurers—have wide latitude to set their own prices, often to the point of what the traffic will bear; and (2) briefly consider how these supply-siders fight against any constraints by government to rein in prices.

EXPLOITIVE PRICING ACROSS THE BOARD

Physicians.

Since physicians order almost all health care services that are delivered, we'll start here. Right away we see a picture of minimal constraints of fee-setting and widespread conflicts of interest. Marc A. Rodwin, Professor of Law at Suffolk University Law School, has this to say about the role of physicians in his book *Medicine, Money & Morals: Physicians' Conflicts of Interest*:

"Traditionally, medical culture has encouraged physicians to act in the best interests of patients. But today, the lure of incentives promotes financially driven conduct, deflecting this intent.... American society's failure to face physicians' conflicts of interest squarely had led to major distortions in the way medicine is practiced, compromised the loyalty of doctors to patients, and resulted in harm to individual patients, society, and the integrity of the medical profession. Today, medicine, money and morals are often in dangerous conflict." [3]

Looking at how physicians' fees are set exposes a process conducive to more self-interest and conflicts of interest than meet the eye. Reimbursement rates for health care services have been set by physicians' organizations since the 1950s with the advent of the relative value scale by the California Medical Association. Further refined in later years as the resource-based relative value scale (RBRVS), it has long favored surgical and diagnostic procedural services over primary care services. The fee-for-service (FFS) system of reimbursement has encouraged many physicians to increase their volume of procedural services, often beyond clear-cut indications of their necessity.

A major mechanism of setting fees is that of the American Medical Association, which convenes its Relative Value Scale Update Committee (RUC) three times a year to recommend valuations for billing codes. The 29 members are mostly selected by medical specialty societies, with very little representation of primary care specialties. RUC's recommendations are generally followed by the Center for Medicare and Medicaid Services (CMS), involving the allocation of some $525 million in annual Medicare spending. As expected, each specialty society has an interest in gaining maximal reimbursement for its services, so that some of its recommendations are way out of line (e.g. a billing code allowing podiatrists to "earn" more than $3,100 by treating a foot ulcer with the skin substitute Dermagraft). Although CMS is aware of overvalued billing codes, it lacks the authority to correct the problem. As William Hsiao, professor of economics at the Harvard School of Public Health, observes:

"You do not turn this over to the people who have a strong interest in the outcome. Every society only wants its specialty's value to go up... You cannot avoid its potential conflict." [4]

A 2008 study documented that physician fees are major contributors to health care costs, and are much higher than physician fees in comparison countries, particularly fees for specialists. As one example, compared to their counterparts in six other OECD countries, U.S. orthopedic surgeons are paid 70 percent more for hip replacements by public payers and 120 percent more by private payers. Public payments for uncomplicated initial hip replacement surgery ranged from $652 in Canada to $1,634 in the U.S., while private health insurance payments were almost $4,000 in the U.S., almost double the private rate in the other countries.[5]

Pharmaceutical Industry.

Over most of the last 25 years, the pharmaceutical industry has been the most profitable industry in the country. Since we have all come to know how expensive prescription drugs can be, pricing practices have come under considerable scrutiny for many years.

In her classic book *The Truth About the Drug Companies: How They Deceive Us and What to Do About It*, Dr. Marcia Angell, former editor of *The New England Journal of Medicine*, exposes how exploitive this industry's pricing practices are. As is only good business practice, drug companies are always seeking the next "blockbuster" drugs, and when found, charging what the traffic will bear. Recent years have seen a growing number of specialty drugs called biologics, mostly for cancer, often with costs up to $100,000 a year. Such costs have led payers, whether insurers or employers, to set limits on what they will pay for these drugs, while making them increasingly unaffordable for patients.

The drug industry has consistently argued (and lobbied hard) that its prices are required if it is to continue to bring innovative drugs to market. As Dr. Angell recounts its usual arguments:

> "Yes, prescription drugs are expensive, but that shows how valuable they are. Besides, our research and development costs are enormous, and we need to cover them somehow. As 'research-based' companies, we turn out a steady stream of innovative medicines that lengthen life, enhance its quality, and avert more expensive health care. You are the beneficiaries of this ongoing achievement of our American free enterprise system, so be grateful, quit whining, and pay up."[6]

Yet the facts tell another story, as these findings document:[7]

- About 85 percent of the industry's products are not innovative, and are merely "me too" drugs, with a slight change in its structure intended to replace a drug that is going off patent.[8]
- About one-half of the largest drug companies are based in Europe (the exact number changes with mergers). This shows that drug companies can still make money in publicly financed systems, including profits necessary to fuel innovation.
- As Schering-Plough's top-selling allergy drug, Claritin approached the end of its patent, its price was raised 13 times over five years, by more than 50 percent overall, more than four times the rate of inflation.
- While drug companies claim to spend an average of $1.3 billon on R & D to bring out a new drug, an exhaustive 2011 study has found that number to be more like $98 million in U.S. dollars; 84 percent of the R & D costs of new drugs is paid for from public sources, mainly the National Institutes of Health.[9]

Studies of drug prices in markets overseas compared to the U.S. also reveal gaming of markets to maximize profits, while clouding their pricing strategies with disinformation. *Price discrimination* is the term used within the industry to describe the process of setting prices from one country to another. The industry acknowledges that drugs are priced higher in the U.S., again arguing that manufacturers have to recover their high R & D costs. Their prices are lower in Europe and Canada where governments exert more pressure to hold down prices. As one example, a one-month supply of Lipitor (excluding mark-up and dispensing fees) averages $129.00 in the U.S. In Canada, the cost is $31.00, in France just $0.43.[10] Antivenom for treating the sting of a bark scorpion gives us another even more striking example of price gouging in this country. The drug—Anascorp, has been available in Mexico for years at a cost of about $100 a dose. Across the border in Arizona, it is priced to patients at $12,000 per dose, and a full treatment with multiple doses can cost up to $50,000. The drug company sells the drug to another firm for $3,500 per dose, which passes it along to hospitals for about $3,780.[11-]

A 2011 study has found that drug pricing in rich countries is relatively unrestrained, since insurance coverage often makes patients insensitive to price. It also found that drug companies tend to charge what higher-income consumers can pay, recognizing that many middle and lower-income people cannot afford them.[12] Out-of-pocket expenditures are increasing as drug costs keep accelerating and as employers and insurers take steps to shift more costs to patients.

A vignette shows how devastating these abstract prices can be for sick patients, even when insured, in this "rich" country.

> *Judy Ariba had her cancer drug for promyelocytic leukemia jump from $10 to $1,700 a month after a long hospital stay and chemotherapy. The monthly cost of the drug Tretinoin is $6,800, but her employer imposed a new 25 percent co-insurance payment at that time. As Judy said 'No one has $1,700 a month.... Now I will get sicker and die.'* [13]

While the drug industry claims to vary its prices based on income levels of other countries, another recent study contradicts this claim. It analyzed drug prices in 14 middle-income countries, such as Brazil, Egypt, Mexico, Poland and South Africa, and compared these with three high-income countries (the U.S., the U.K. and France). The study also compared prices in middle-income countries with low-income countries such as Cameroon, Guinea and Republic of Congo. They found that some middle-income countries actually pay more for drugs than high-income countries, and that other middle-income countries pay prices below those in low-income countries.[14] The import of this is clear: charge more in countries where patients lack clout and have little protection from government—all in keeping with the profit drive of the free market.

The drug industry fiercely defends its pricing prerogative and for many years has successfully fended off any price controls by the U.S. government. Through lobbying and campaign spending, it got what it wanted (new subsidized markets) with the 2003 Medicare Prescription Drug, Improvement, and Modernization Act (MMA) and in the 2010 Patient Protection and Affordable Care Act (ACA) (no importation of drugs from Canada and other countries, no price controls and more subsidized patients). All that leaves us with the highest costs of drugs in the world, with only one card that can make them more affordable—the Canada Frequent Visitor card. (Figure 4.1)

FIGURE 4.1

Bargains For Drugs

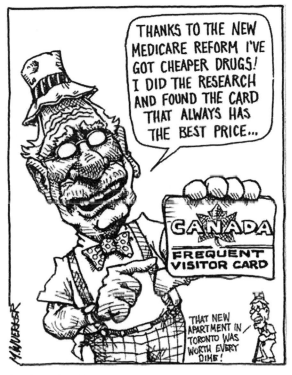

Copyright by Matt Wuerker.

Source: Reprinted with permission from Matt Wuerker

Hospitals.

U.S. hospitals have by far the highest prices in the world. How they set their prices is completely undecipherable to almost all of us. It has been described by Princeton University's economist Uwe Reinhardt as "chaos behind a wall of secrecy." Karen Davis, president of the Commonwealth Fund, gives us these insights:

- Nonprofit hospitals charge patients less than for-profit hospitals (including effective net prices after discounts).

- Nonprofit hospitals admit more uninsured patients and provide more uncompensated care than for-profit hospitals.
- Prices bear little relationship to the actual cost of care. Some specialized services, such as burn units and neonatal intensive care are "money losers"; others, such as cardiac surgery and radiological imaging services, are highly profitable.
- Pricing, uncompensated care, and bill collection practices vary widely across nonprofit hospitals. As a result, the burden of caring for patients who cannot pay is unevenly borne; academic medical centers, as teaching hospitals, take on a larger responsibility for uncompensated care than community hospitals.
- The financial stability of hospitals varies widely. Some are in serious financial difficulty, others are on the margin, and others are doing well. Hospitals in the best position are not the best quality or the most efficient, while those doing the worst are largely shouldering a disproportionate share of charity care.
- The cost per day [of hospital care] is three times the OECD median country cost per day, and the cost per capita is twice the OECD median country.
- [Compared to other goods and services, key differences of hospital care] include   lack of information, limited choice, complexity and life-critical importance of health care treatment decisions, physicians' decision-making role, and the need for insurance to protect financial security.[15] (These differences, of course, also apply to other transactions by patients with the health care system.)

Commissioned by the California Nurses Association, a 2004 study by the Institute for Health and Socio-Economic Policy (IHSP) of more than 4,100 U.S. hospitals found huge markups in charges to patients, especially for prescription drugs, medical supplies, and surgical procedures. The country's 100 most expensive hospitals marked up their gross charges by an average of 673 percent (not a typo!) over their costs, or $673.00 for a patient's bill when the costs were $100.00. The "leading" hospital in medical supply markups charged an astounding $9,593 for supplies costing $100.00, while the "leader" for prescription drugs charged $6,796 for drugs costing $100.00! For-profit hospitals had an average sticker price marked up by 351 percent over costs, while government hospitals had the lowest average markups at 185 percent over costs.[16]

Figure 4.2 shows how wide these markups can be among hospitals in California.[17] Not shown is an even bigger over-charger, Memorial Hospital in Redding, CA, a member of Tenet Healthcare, the second largest investor-owned hospital chain, which was found in a 2002 report to be charging *ten* times state averages for drugs.[18]

FIGURE 4.2

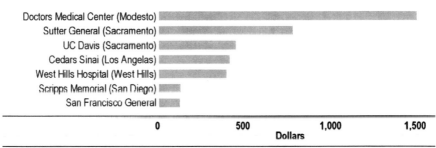

Charges For a Chest X-Ray at
Selected California Hospitals, 2004

Source: Reprinted with permission from Lagnado, L. California hospitals open books, showing huge price differences. *Wall Street Journal*, December 27, 2004.

In a important article in 2006, Uwe Reinhardt explained as clearly as humanly possible how hospitals set their prices and get paid. But as he notes, William McGowan, chief financial officer of the University of California, Davis, Health System with 30 years' experience in hospital financing, readily admits: "There is no method to this madness. As we went through the years, we had these cockamamie formulas. We multiplied our costs to set our charges."

Suffice to say, for our purposes here, that hospital financing is an extremely complex business. As in the drug industry, we again encounter price discrimination, whereby hospitals charge different payers different prices for identical health care services. Self-paying uninsured patients receive the highest bills, insurers try to negotiate down hospital prices as much as possible, and government payers have their own, often changing formulas that hospitals see as underpayments. Medicare accounts for about one-third of hospital revenues through flat payments per hospital case for some 750 diagnostic related groups (DRGs), while private insurers account for another one-third (often with discounts of 50 percent or more).[19]

To be fair, there is no question that hospitals have a difficult time dealing with our unstable and dysfunctional health care system. Some of the variables include case mix, regional costs, type of hospital, and demography of the population being served. But at the same time, there is unquestionably price gouging going on by many hospitals, especially for-profit hospitals, which tend to abandon their locations when not sufficiently profitable.

It could logically be argued that adding regulations imposes further costs, driving prices still higher. But in the state that regulates its hospitals most heavily, there is an important lesson. Maryland regulates its hospitals more than any other state, and yet had the lowest state average markups on charges over costs in 2004, an average of 120 percent. Counter to the argument that regulation impedes financial stability, two-thirds of its hospitals are still profitable (right on the national average).[20]

The latest trend among hospitals is an arms race in expanding existing ERs and building new free-standing ERs. On the surface, this might seem like an example of free markets competing to deliver better care by building their capacity, perhaps even lowering costs to patients. But this unfortunately is far from the case. Not only do these ER networks expand into affluent areas with well-insured patients, they are intended to build referrals to their base hospitals and become cash cows themselves. Blurring the lines between what are really emergency problems, these ERs typically charge three or four times what equivalent services would have cost in primary care clinics or urgent care centers (e.g. $700 for a sprained ankle). In Washington State, where this is a growing trend, state Senator Karen Keiser, chair of the Senate Health & Long-Term Care Committee, has this to say:

> "It's alarming because increasing emergency-room use pushes costs but doesn't improve care. They're totally countering what we're trying to accomplish: improving access and containing cost."[21]

Thus the build-out of ERs increases costs, even as it increases supply, by moving patients away from lower-cost care with primary care physicians and urgent care clinics to high-cost ER interventions. In this instance, despite ideological claims that competition lowers costs, competition and costs rise together.

When all is said and done, and despite all the protestations of the hospital industry that they are "barely making it." Figure 4.3 shows how far out of line U.S. hospitals are for average cost per hospital stay compared to other nations.[22] Table 4.1 lists big differences in hospital charges for three common services in the U.S, France and Canada.[23]

FIGURE 4.3

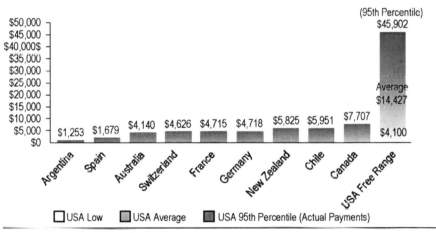

Average Cost Per Hospital Stay in Selected Countries ($U.S.)

Source: Reprinted with permission from International Federation of Health Plans, 2010 Comparative Price Report. Medical and Hospital Fees by Country, p 24

Insurers.

Private insurers are experts at hiking their premiums and giving us less in return.

They keep blaming providers and hospitals as the main drivers of health care inflation. While they are correct in much of this, they refuse to accept their own big contribution to health care costs. As is argued in detail in my 2008 book, *Do Not Resuscitate: Why the Health Insurance Industry Is Dying, and How We Must Replace It*, we can no longer afford the private health insurance industry.

TABLE 4.1

Hospital Charges For Scans and Imaging Fees in U.S. Dollars

	FRANCE	CANADA	UNITED STATES
CT Scan of Abdomen	$179	$61	$164 to $1,564
CT Scan of Head	$179	$65	$82 to $1,430
MRI Scan	$398	$304	$509 to $2,590

Source: International Federation of Health Plans. 2010 Comparative Price Report. Medical and Hospital Fees by Country. October 2010

According to the Milliman Medical Index, the total cost of health care (premiums plus out-of-pocket costs) for a family of four in an employer-sponsored preferred provider plan (PPO) in 2011 was more than $19,000, toward which employees paid an average of $4,728 in premiums and $3,280 in out-of-pocket costs.[24] There is no relief in sight—in a survey of 1,700 firms, PricewaterhouseCoopers estimates that premiums will rise by 8.5 percent in 2012.[25]

As we saw in chapter 4, the nation's five largest for-profit health insurers netted $11.7 billion in profits in 2010, up from 51 percent in 2008, even as many insured patients skimped on medical care to avoid co-pays and deductibles. Profits rose by 361 percent at Cigna from 2008 to 2010.[26,27]Meanwhile, health insurers were pushing for double-digit premium increases (some as high as 39 to 50 percent!).

Private insurers have been quite candid about their real goal: profits and shareholder return over service to enrollees. In 2008, WellPoint's CEO Angela Braly assured analysts that her company would "not sacrifice profitability for membership." More recently, as the recession continues without end in sight, Aetna's CFO Joseph Zubretsky said much the same thing: "We would like to have both profit and growth, but if you have to choose between one or the other, you take margin and profit and you sacrifice the growth line." [28] These statements clearly illustrate the main goal of these companies—profits before service, as is their obligation to shareholders.

Insurers have many ways to glean profits from enrollees, and are especially adept at cherry-picking the market for healthier enrollees and denying claims when they get sick. These are just some of the ways that they build profits at our expense:

- Deny coverage at the outset, or if covered, deny claims.
- Bait and switch—attract enrollees with lower premiums, then sequentially raise premiums, especially for enrollees with claims.
- Cancel policies for an entire group, or withdraw from the market.
- Restrict enrollees to limited networks of hospitals and providers, with higher cost sharing for going out of network and for tiered prescription drugs.
- Increase cost-sharing, including higher deductibles, in both private and privatized Medicare and Medicaid plans.
- Offer "mini-med" policies that hardly qualify as insurance, some with annual limits of what the insurer will cover (as low as $2,000).

Much as the insurance industry complains about regulation, it remains under-regulated. Most oversight is at the state level, and most states have relatively lax requirements. Insurers often game this by locating their headquarters in states with lax oversight and selling policies across state lines. Some states, such as California, have the authority to review rate increases in advance, but not to block them. As an example, even though an increase of 16 percent by Anthem Blue Cross was considered "unreasonable" by California regulators, the rate increase went ahead anyway.[29] The Affordable Care Act will not set up more intensive regulation until 2014 when health insurance exchanges are put in place. Until then the federal government has limited authority to restrain rate increases, even though it will review rate increases in excess of 10 percent. An interesting new development as of this writing is a lawsuit brought by Anthem Health Plans of Maine arguing that state regulators violated state law and the U.S. Constitution by reducing their rate increases in the previous three years. This case will be closely followed by other insurers, and may have national industry-wide implications.[30]

HOW SUPPLY SIDE STAKEHOLDERS FIGHT PRICE RESTRAINTS—AND WIN!

As we saw in the last chapter, competition doesn't work well in health care. Instead, corporate stakeholder economic and political power tends to carry the day. Each sector in the health care industry may work separately to best meet its own self-interest. In other instance, sectors may have common interests and work together to fend off regulation. One example is the cooperative efforts of the insurance and drug industries in passing the 2003 Medicare drug bill (MMA), which brings handsome profits to both industries, working through three senior non-profit groups—the United Seniors Association, the Seniors Coalition and 60 Plus, and America 21.[31] These are all conservative groups, free market-oriented, and in the case of America 21, a conservative Christian group. Another is the support of physician organizations for insurers' efforts to avoid rate-setting regulations, since physicians fear that their fees will be cut as a consequence of any insurance rate reduction.[32]

The power of the medical-industrial complex is telling when we see how closely Wall Street follows corporate stakeholders and how the stock market reacts to changes in health care legislation. In 2009, for example, health care stocks rose more than 28 percent in less than three months after Congress released the first of its health care bills, which included no significant price controls.[33] In the buildup to the Affordable Care Act, trading in UnitedHealthcare and WellPoint jumped by three-fold as traders placed new calls and puts within hours after the Obama Administration signaled its willingness to look at options replace or kill the public option; health care stocks were pushed higher even as the broader market suffered a triple-digit loss.[34]

Supply-side stakeholders have a full quiver of arrows to influence public opinion and policy in their favor. Here are some examples across several industries:

- As the battle was being waged in Congress in 2009, Regence BlueCross BlueShield ran a slick campaign on the Internet, social media and billboards blaming patients for much of the blame for high health insurance premiums.[35]
- WellPoint gave $842,000 to the Republican State Leadership Committee for the 2010 elections, and was a major donor to

Republican organizations in the Wisconsin recall elections in 2011.[36]

- One stealth strategy used by the drug industry is to finance charity organizations which then turn around and pay co-payments for expensive drugs for patients unable to afford them; it's good PR, and drug companies also gain by the increased sales while deducting their charitable donations.[37]
- In the aftermath of the U.S. Supreme Court's ruling in 2011 that drug marketing is protected as free speech under the First Amendment, drug companies are now lobbying to end rules by the FDA against marketing off-label use of prescription drugs.[38]
- People associated with venture capital funds that underwrite medical devices and other health products have made more than $3 million in political donations over the last five years to politicians on both sides of the aisle and to political action committees; the National Venture Capital Association, a lobbying group for the medical device industry, has targeted its efforts at easing regulation of the industry.[39]

Returning to the aforementioned classic 2003 *Health Affairs* paper, I find this description to be spot-on in explaining how all this works; it is just as accurate today as then:

"In the U.S. system, money flows from households to the providers of health care through a vast network of relatively uncoordinated pipes and capillaries of various sizes. Although the huge federal Medicare program and the federal-state Medicaid programs do possess some monopsonistic purchasing power, and large private insurers may enjoy some degree of monopsony power as well in some localities, the highly fragmented buy side of the U.S. health system is relatively weak by international standards. It is one factor, among others, that could explain the relatively high prices paid for health care and for health professionals in the United States."[40]

Even though prices are a big part of our problem in our runaway health care non-system, there are other important culprits at work. As we will soon see in the next chapter, as stakeholders gain market share through consolidation, health care costs go up, not down.

References

1. Anderson, GE, Reinhardt, UE, Hussery, PS, Petrosyan, V. It's the prices, stupid: Why the United States is so different from other countries. *Health Affairs* 22 (3): 89-105, 2003.
2. Organization for Economic Cooperation and Development (OECD). *Health at a Glance 2011: OECD Indicators.* November 23, 2011.
3. Rodwin, MA. *Medicine, Money, and Morals: Physicians' Conflicts of Interest.* New York. Oxford University Press, 1993, p. 247.
4. Matthews, AW. Secrets of the system: Physician panel prescribes the fees paid by Medicare. *Wall Street Journal*, October 27, 2010: A1.
5. Laugesen, MJ, Glied, SA. Higher fees paid to U.S. physicians drive higher spending for physician services compared to other countries. *Health Affairs* 30 (9): 1647-56, 2011.
6. Angell, M. The Truth About the Drug Companies. *New York Review of Books*, July 15, 2004.
7. Ibid # 6.
8. Light, DW. (ed).*The Risk of Prescription Drugs*. New York. Columbia University Press, 2010.
9. Light, DW, Warburton, R. Demythologizing the high costs of pharmaceutical research. *BioSocieties*, 2011, pp 1-17.
10. International Federation of Health Plans. 2010 Comparative Price Report. Medical and Hospital Fees by Country, p 24.
11. Gold, J. Treating a scorpion sting: $100 in Mexico or $12,000 in U.S. *Kaiser Health News*, November 28, 2011.
12. Danzon, PM, Towse, A, Mulcahy, AW. Setting cost-effectiveness thresholds as a means to achieve appropriate drug prices in rich and poor countries. *Health Affairs* 30 (8): 1529-38, 2011.
13. Appleby, J. Some employers make patients pay a percentage of cost instead of a co-pay. *Kaiser Health News*, August 22, 2011.
14. Morel, CM, McGuire, A, Mossialos, E. The level of income appears to have no consistent bearing on pharmaceutical prices across countries. *Health Affairs* 30 (8): 1545-52, 2011.
15. Davis, K. Hospital pricing behavior and patient financial risk. New York. The Commonwealth Fund, June 22, 2004.
16. Senior Journal. Study of 4,000 U.S. hospitals shows high hospital charges fuel national healthcare crisis; names most, least expensive. September 10, 2004. Available at http://senior journal.com/NEWS/Features/4-09-10Hospitals.htm
17. Lagnado, L. California hospitals open books, showing huge price differences. *Wall Street Journal*, December 27, 2004.

18. Abelson, R. Nurses' Association says in study that big hospital chain overcharges patients for drugs. *New York Times*, November 24, 2002.
19. Reinhardt, UE. The pricing of U.S. hospital services: Chaos behind a wall of secrecy. *Health Affairs* 25 (1): 57-69, 2006.
20. Ibid # 16.
21. Ostrom, CM. ER building boom is wrong prescription, critics say. *The Seattle Times*, November 27, 2011.
22. Ibid # 10, p. 10.
23. Ibid # 10, pp. 5,6,8.
24. McCanne, D. The Milliman Medical Index ($19,393) in perspective. May 12, 2011. Available at www.pnhp.org/blog
25. Goozner, M. *The Fiscal Times*, May 18, 2011.
26. Health insurers pocketed huge profits in 2010 despite weak economy. Health Care for America Now, March 3, 2011.
27. Abelson, R. Health insurers making record profits as many postpone care. *New York Times*, May 13, 2011.
28. Potter, W. Fresh evidence that insurance companies value profits over people. *Huffington Post*, August 1, 2011.
29. Appleby, J. States face challenges in controlling health insurance premiums. *Kaiser Health News*, August 7, 2011.
30. Appleby, J. Big insurer fights back in court against regulation of profit margin. *Kaiser Health News*, October 31, 2011.
31. Dreyfuss, BT. Poison pill: How Abramoff's cronies sold the Medicare drug bill. *The Washington Monthly* 38 (11): 23-9, November 2006.
32. Ibid # 29.
33. Hamsher, J. Fact sheet: The truth about the health care bill. FireDogLake, March 19, 2010.
34. Tracy, T. UnitedHealth, Aetna, WellPoint get bullish signal. *Wall Street Journal*, August 18, 2009: C3.
35. Beebe, P. Regence campaign: Consumers must make choices to reduce health care costs. *The Salt Lake Tribune*, November 14, 2009.
36. Salant. WellPoint joins Koch help fight Wisconsin state senate recalls. Bloomberg.com, August 4, 2011.
37. Anand, G. Support system: Through charities, drug makers help people—and themselves. *Wall Street Journal*, December 1, 2005: A1.
38. Burton, TM. The free speech pill: Drug firms see opening to push for end to off-label marketing ban. *Wall Street Journal*, November 3, 20-11: B1.
39. Meier, B, Roberts, J. Venture capitalists put money on easing medical device rules. New York Times, October 25, 2011. Available at http://www.nytimes.com/2011/10/26/business/venture-capitalist
40. Ibid # 1, p.102.

The Promise:
**LARGER MARKET SHARE BRINGS COSTS DOWN
AND IMPROVES SERVICE**

CHAPTER 5

Consolidation and Market Power: Another Theory Bites The Dust

We have seen how competition in health care markets doesn't bring down prices or costs, while also tending not to add to value of services delivered. But how about consolidation among stakeholders? Will they perform better if they have a larger market share?

In this chapter we will (1) answer that question by looking at four major players in the medical-industrial complex—insurers, hospitals, nursing homes, and PhRMA; and (2) briefly discuss the changing political dynamics among these stakeholders as the provisions of the Patient Protection and Affordable Care Act (ACA) of 2010 approach possible implementation.

CONSOLIDATION AND DIVERSIFICATION ON THE SUPPLY SIDE

Insurance Industry

The five largest health insurers are on a buying spree, acquiring companies in health information technology, physician management, and other related industries that will give them more clout and market share to shape the delivery system. While they couch their intent in an effort to contain health care costs, they are paying close attention to increasing their already well-paid financial bottom lines.

These examples give a sense of the frenetic activity among the largest five insurers in an effort to expand their holdings and roles in the health care marketplace: [1]

- United HealthGroup, the $100 billion behemoth and the largest insurer by revenue, already sells technology to hospitals, distributes prescription drugs, manages clinical trials, and offers continuing medical education. In 2009, its subsidiary Ingenix acquired AIM Healthcare, the leading data mining and insurance claim auditing service in the country. Now it is moving into the purchase of medical groups and starting physician management companies. United's subsidiary, OptumHealth, operates a Collaborative Care unit that recently launched Lifeprint, a physician network serving United's private Medicare plans. United HealthGroup has also purchased the management arm of Monarch HealthCare, an association based in Irvine, California with some 2,300 physicians in a range of specialties.[2]
- A 2004 merger between Anthem and WellPoint Health Networks made it the largest insurer in the country in terms of number of lives covered. The Indianapolis-based giant operates a large number of Blue Cross Blue Shield plans in many states around the country. In 2011, WellPoint acquired CareMore, a health plan operator with a network of 26 clinics in California, Arizona and Nevada that focus on preventive care and the care of some 54,000 chronically ill seniors enrolled in Medicare Advantage plans in the Los Angeles area with 26 clinics.[3]
- CIGNA has an expanding medical group in the Phoenix area with 32 locations. In late 2011 it bought the Medicare carrier HealthSpring Inc. for $3.8 billion, thereby gaining a major source of Medicare prescription drug plans and Medicare Advantage enrollees.[4]
- Humana spent almost $800 million to acquire Concentra, a chain that runs urgent- and occupational-care clinics in some 40 states, and employs about 1,000 primary care physicians who live close to where 3 million Humana enrollees live.[5]
- Aetna is partnering with Carilion Clinic in Virginia to build an accountable care organization (ACO) in advance of the ACA bringing ACOs on line in 2014; Aetna has also bought Prodigy Health Holdings for $600 million in order to provide mid-size companies with a self-funded insurance option.[6]

All of these actions toward increasing consolidation have had a number of adverse consequences, as these examples document:

- The UnitedHealth story is one of unvarnished greed at the highest level in the company. Dr. William McGuire, pulmonologist, CEO and chairman of United Health for 15 years, was forced to resign in 2006 following investigations by the SEC, IRS and U.S. Attorney's office into stock options backdating. It was shown that he picked past dates for his options awards when share prices were lower, then signed papers as if he were granted the options on that earlier date, thereby increasing the options' values. As an article in his local newspaper reported: "'Dollar Bill' has made lots of news with cash-and-stock paydays that have topped $100 million in recent years—and he's still sittting atop stock options valued at $1.6 billion. McGuire's admiring outside board members—10 of whom have become millionaires through the sale of their own appreciated stock in recent years—have defended his league-leading compensation on grounds that the giant health insurer's stock price has been a superb performer."[7]

  As the scandal ended up, McGuire agreed to repay $468 million as a partial settlement of the backdating prosecution, including giving back $320 million in stock options, forgoing more than $99 million in other retirement and executive savings benefits, and settling a $7 million civil penalty.[8]

- In 2010, when UnitedHealth had built a strong lobbying capacity for legislation favorable to itself ($1.8 spending on lobbying through seven different lobbying firms and another $1 million through its own corporate PAC called "United for Health" that year), it received a 65 percent unfavorable rating in a survey of hospital executives.[9]

- A 2010 report by the AMA, *Competition in Health Insurance: A Comprehensive Study of U.S Markets*, found that 99 percent of 313 metropolitan areas tracked would be considered to have "highly concentrated" markets under the guidelines used by the U.S. Department of Justice and the Federal Trade Commission.[10]

- Over the first year after passage of the ACA, shares of the six largest health insurers gained an average of 16 percent on Wall Street, better than all other multiple-company sectors in health care.[11]

- Wall Street analysts note that insurance industry profit margins have historically averaged 7 to 8 percent, and expect that number to drop to 5 percent or lower when medical loss requirements are implemented by ACA. In response, the above new directions are expected to bring much higher returns. United HealthGroup's initiative in information technology has realized profit margins above 20 percent in the past, and is projected to be about 14 percent in 2011.[12]

- A 2011 report by Goldman Sachs researchers stated that Medicare enrollees are worth more than any other category of enrollee in a merger or acquisition deal. By their calculations, Medicare Advantage enrollees have a "value per member" of $6,000 in such a deal, compared to $1,500 for members of employer-based plans and $1,200 for Medicaid beneficiaries.[13]

- A longer view of these trends is provided by a 2010 study which examined a proprietary dataset of employer-sponsored health plans covering more than 10 million Americans annually between 1998 and 2006. The report concludes that "consolidation facilitates the exercise of monopsonistic power *vis a vis* physicians, whose absolute employment and relative earnings decline in its wake."[14]

- A 2011 study by the Commonwealth Fund examined state trends in insurance premiums and deductibles from 2003 to 2010. It found that the three largest private insurers controlled more than 70 percent of the market in 24 states, and more than 80 percent in 10 states plus the District of Columbia. (Figure 5.1) This study also found that 62 percent of the U.S. population lives in states where total premiums accounted for 20 percent or more than of middle incomes! (Figure 5.2) [15]

Hospital Industry

The U.S. hospital industry is much bigger, more diverse and fractionated than most of us realize. No longer is there the long-standing hospital in the center of the community that our parents knew and where we may have been born. Today the industry is complex and torn between its business interests and traditional service role. There has been an accelerating trend for physicians to shift their practices to ambulatory facilities and to specialty hospitals focused on only certain well-reimbursed services, such as cardiac care and orthopedic surgery.

FIGURE 5.1

Market Share of Three Largest Health Insurers, by State, 2010

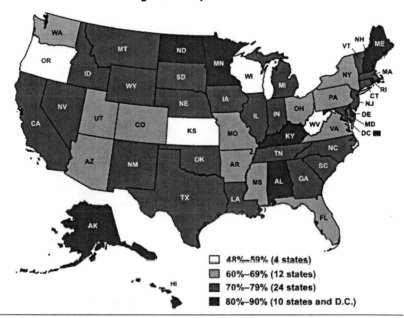

48%–59% (4 states)
60%–69% (12 states)
70%–79% (24 states)
80%–90% (10 states and D.C.)

Hospitals have long struggled with how to continue money-losing services (e.g. psychiatric services). They have survived by cost-shifting to payers that can pay higher prices. But as their prices continue to escalate, that strategy becomes less and less effective in staying afloat.

Another strategy for dealing with care that loses money is to abandon it, as has been done by specialty hospitals. They are for-profit and investor-owned (often by physicians practicing there), and give up other service obligations, including emergency rooms.

Much of the industry is now driven more by the business "ethic" than its traditional service mission. These examples show how the bigger, investor-owned players increasingly dominate the industry and raise prices in their quest to satisfy investors:

- HCA, the nation's largest hospital chain, was bought out by three private equity firms on Wall Street in 2001 for $31.6 billion in the biggest leveraged buyout in U.S. history.[16] When HCA Holdings

FIGURE 5.2

Employer Premiums as Percentage of Median Household Income for Under-65 Population, 2003 and 2010

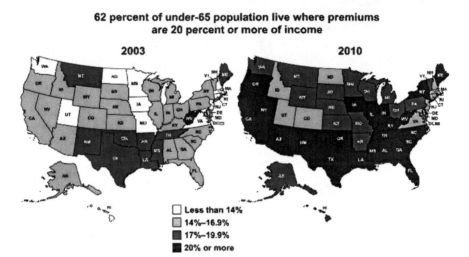

62 percent of under-65 population live where premiums
are 20 percent or more of income

☐ Less than 14%
▨ 14%–16.9%
▨ 17%–19.9%
■ 20% or more

Sources: 2003 and 2010 Medical Expenditure Panel Survey–Insurance Component (for total average premiums for employer-based
health insurance plans. weighted by single and family household distribution): 2003–04 and 2009–10 Current Population Surveys
(for median household incomes for under-65 population).

went public in 2011, their owners had paid themselves about
$4.3 billion in dividends over the previous year (almost that of
their original investment), and were each expecting a profit of
about $3 billion from their original $1.2 billion investment.[17]

- In its periodic Community Tracking Study of 12 nationally
  representative communities across the country, the Center for
  Studying Health System Change has concluded that "specialty
  hospitals are contributing to a medical arms race that is driving
  up costs without demonstrating clear quality advantages."[18]

- Non-profit hospitals, including those owned by state and local
  governments, account for about 80 percent of U.S. hospitals,
  according to the American Hospital Association. But their
  numbers are dwindling fast due to falling reimbursement,
  declining operating margins, and growth in mergers.[19]

- Between 1990 and 2009, the number of hospital emergency
  rooms in non-rural areas declined by 27 percent; low-margin,
  for profit facilities were the most likely to close their ERs.[20]

- The more consolidated hospitals become in communities, the more they hire physicians under productivity-based contractual terms. These contracts reward physicians for ordering more expensive tests and providing a higher volume of services. The latest trend is for hospitals to employ more primary care physicians in an effort to increase their referrals and market share. Costs go up in two ways—by doing more than is appropriate or necessary, and by hospitals charging facility fees, even when the employed physicians remain in their own offices but are now under contract to a hospital.[21] A flagrant example of exorbitant facility fees is demonstrated by a mother taking her 4-year-old son to see a dermatologist in an outpatient office on the SSM Cardinal Glennon Children's Medical Center campus in St. Louis. Several weeks after a 3-minute procedure to treat her son's warts, she received a bill for $538 ($220 for the physician and $318 for the hospital's facility fee).[22]

Nursing Homes

The nursing home world is one of big corporate business—much bigger than most of us are aware. A 2011 study of the ownership, financing and management strategies of the 10 largest for-profit nursing home chains in the U.S. gives us an overview of the industry. Of the almost 16,000 nursing homes in the country, 70 percent are for-profit and 54 percent are controlled by corporate chains. HCR Manor Care, Toledo, OH, the largest of the 10 corporate chains, has 278 nursing homes in 30 states, a total of 38,140 beds, 60,000 employees, and $4 billion in operating revenue. In 2007, it was purchased for $6.6 billion by Carlyle Group, a global private equity firm with more than $85 billion in equity capital in 64 funds. Both private companies and publicly held chains have complex organizational structures with multiple investors, holding companies, and multiple levels of ownership, in part to insulate the parent companies from liability. As the researchers conclude in their 2011 report:

"The chains have used strategies to maximize shareholder and investor value that include increasing Medicare revenues, occupancy rates, and company diversification, establishing multiple layers of corporate ownership, developing real estate investment trusts, and creating limited liability companies. These strategies enhance shareholder and investor profits, reduce corporate taxes, and reduce liability risk. There is a need for greater transparency in ownership and financial reporting and for more government oversight of the largest for-profit chains, including those owned by private equity companies.[23]

An important follow-up study in 2012 documented that the quality of care in for-profit nursing home chains is much worse than in their not-for-profit counterparts, and is a serious threat to seniors' care, as these findings show:

- Lower staffing, especially for RNs, even below recommended minimum staffing levels.
- Despite having sicker patients, nursing hours are 30 percent lower than for non-profit and government nursing homes.
- 36 percent more deficiencies and 41 percent more serious deficiencies (e.g. failure to prevent pressure sores, falls, infections, resident mistreatment).
- The largest for-profit chains purchased by private equity companies between 2003 and 2008 had *more* deficiencies after being acquired.[24]

Pharmaceutical Industry

In addition to what we've already seen in earlier chapters about the drug industry, there is a whole other dimension of the industry that has everything to do with its impacts on costs, choice and quality of service to patients. Pharmacy benefit managers (PBMs), by negotiating prices for drugs and the rates that pharmacies will be reimbursed, act as middlemen between drug companies, pharmacies and their customers, which include insurers, employers and other groups. The 2011 merger of the country's two largest PBMs, Express Scripts and Medco Health Solutions Inc., gives us a window through which to see how things really work within the industry.

The two rivals agreed to a $29.1 billion merger, subject to regulatory review, that will give the new St. Louis-based firm, Express Scripts Holding Company, control over about one-third of the market for pharmacy benefits, nearly four billion prescriptions each year. One factor in this move was the loss of Medco's contract with UnitedHealth Group, which has tasked its own unit, OptumRx, with managing pharmacy benefits for its enrollees. This is all part of a response by major players in the industry to cut costs, increase their leverage in negotiating with suppliers and customers, and boost their profits.[25]

It remains to be seen whether this big merger and consolidation within the industry will contain rapidly rising drug costs. The Federal Trade Commission will look hard at how this really works. An already largely non-transparent industry will be further clouded by new rounds of negotiations between drug companies, PBMs, employers, insurers and pharmacies. Representing pharmacists and drug stores, the National Association of Chain Drug Stores and the National Community Pharmacists Association worry that "the merged company will be too big to play fair, and will have immense power to unfairly dominate the market." David Balto, a Washington D.C. antitrust lawyer and former policy director at the FTC, says "the FTC is becoming increasingly skeptical about the level of competition in the PBM market." [26]

One example of battles to come in the dispute between Walgreen, the nation's largest drugstore chain, and Express Scripts Inc., which has some 50 million patients and annual revenue of nearly $45 billion. Beyond filling prescriptions, Walgreen pharmacists offer additional services, such as advising customers about appropriate doses and trying to switch them to generics as cheaper alternatives when possible. They want higher reimbursement than Express Scripts Inc. so far is willing to offer.[27] But their contract negotiations broke down at the start of 2012, forcing millions of patients to go elsewhere to fill some 90 million prescriptions for Express Scripts customers previously filled at Walgreens.[28]

All of this is no surprise. It is entirely predictable since Congress handed over the prescription drug benefit to the private sector with the 2003 Medicare Prescription Drug, Improvement, and Modernization Act (MMA). Instead of decreasing costs and providing more choice for patients, we get higher costs, less choice, and no negotiated drug prices as the government does so effectively for the Veterans Administration and Medicaid.

CHANGING POLITICAL DYNAMICS
UNDER HEALTH CARE "REFORM"

As prices and costs of health care continue to soar way above costs of living and average family incomes, corporate stakeholders keep blaming others while excusing their own contributions to the problem. Insurers argue that hospitals and physicians are overcharging them, and that they have no recourse but to raise premiums. Hospitals point to physicians demanding higher payments, as well as their increasing burden to care for the uninsured and low reimbursement from Medicare and Medicaid. Drug companies keep telling us that they need to maintain their pricing structure in order to bring new drugs to market.

Consolidation among these stakeholders will not help to restrain prices and costs. A remarkable degree of consolidation has already occurred. According to a 2010 report by the AMA, for example, one insurer holds 70 percent or more of the health plan market in 24 or 43 states measured.[29] A 2009 report by the Congressional Research Service, *The Market Structure of the Health Insurance Industry,* drew this conclusion about consolidation in the insurance industry:

"The exercise of market power by firms in concentrated markets generally leads to higher prices and reduced output—high premiums and limited access to health insurance—combined with high profits."[30]

Although our market-based system has demonstrated that it cannot control its costs, the 2010 ACA was a gift to corporate stakeholders. They lobbied hard for industry-friendly provisions, and mostly got what they wanted—32 million more insured people (many with government subsidies), expansion of Medicaid, freedom from price controls, and the opportunity to reposition themselves in new accountable care organizations (ACOs).

The ACO story is one to watch. An ACO is a network of doctors, hospitals and/or insurers that shares financial responsibility for providing care to a large group of patients. Under the provisions of the ACA, the government started receiving and reviewing applications for ACOs in January 2012, and the first ones may start as soon as April

2012. The law requires that an ACO will manage all of the health care needs for 5,000 or more Medicare beneficiaries for at least three years. The law also creates the Pioneer Program, which will allow high-performing systems to keep much of the expected savings in return for taking on more financial risk. The Department of Health and Human Services estimates that ACOs could save as much as $940 million in the first four years, mostly by better integration of care and reducing inappropriate and unnecessary services.[31]

The details of exactly how ACOs will work are still somewhat murky, but insurers and hospitals are already going head to head in an effort to dominate the new system. Both are buying up larger physician groups and building new networks. Insurers are moving beyond the Medicare group to privately insured patients. This leaves physician groups in the middle—will they contract or become employed by one or the other? And how much control will either exert on their practices?

How this will play out for physicians will be interesting. Since FFS payment is still largely in use, many of those employed by hospitals will be under pressure to order more expensive tests and increase the volume of well-reimbursed procedures and services. Physicians who work for insurer-sponsored networks will be under increasing pressure to do less rather than more, while finding themselves in practices where their masters increasingly cut costs and intrude on their clinical decisions.

While ACOs are intended to better integrate care and contain costs, they are unlikely to do so. They will lead to greater consolidation among the three major types of players—hospitals, insurers and physician groups—giving them more clout to negotiate prices. Drs. Steffie Woolhandler and David Himmelstein, internists at Harvard Medical School and cofounders of Physicians for a National Health Program, give us this warning:

"While the term ACO remains at best vaguely defined, the concept is hauntingly similar to the capitated managed care experiment that proved disastrous in the 1990s. In both instances, providers receive a set annual payment to cover the costs of all care, and get to keep whatever they don't spend on patients. The obvious winning strategy – from a business point of view – is to recruit relatively healthy patients, offering luxurious care for the healthy and minimally ill, and subtle cues that those with expensive illness would be better off elsewhere. Neither risk adjustment nor quality monitoring schemes are up to the task of blunting these incentives. An ACO can game risk adjustments by ferreting out additional diagnoses that may be clinically unimportant but would up its capitation payment, and make its outcomes look better as well. . . . In sum, the ACO strategy remains an untested theory for health reform. Considerable experience with similar reforms in the past suggests that this ACO strategy will lead to yet another health policy dead end."[32]

In the next chapter we will see how much bureaucracy, waste and profits in the insurance industry, newly empowered by the ACA, will continue to drive up costs at the expense of patients.

References

1. Weaver, C. Managed care enters the exam room as insurers buy doctor groups. *Washington Post*, July 1, 2011.
2. Mathews, AW. UnitedHealth buys California group of 2,300 doctors. *Wall Street Journal*, September 1, 2011.
3. Mathews, AW, Loftus, P. WellPoint to acquire CareMore. *Wall Street Journal*, June 9, 2011.
4. Mathews, AW, Kamp, J. Cigna to buy Medicare carrier. *Wall Street Journal*, October 25, 2011.
5. Johnson, A. Reforms prod insurers to diversify. *Wall Street Journal*, May 12, 2011.
6. Ibid # 5.
7. St. Anthony, N. McGuire's payday is a shame, if not a crime. Twin Cities *StarTribune* business, April 21, 2006.
8. Thoelcke, T. Money losers of 2007: William McGuire surrenders $600 million, December 23, 2007. Accessed at htpp://www.bloggingstocks.com/2007/12/23/money-losers-of-2...
9. Wikipedia. UnitedHealth Group. Htpp://en.wikipedia.org/wike/UnitedHealth_Group, accessed February 3, 2012.
10. Berry, E. Health plans extend their market dominance. *American Medical News*, March 8, 2010.
11. Britt, R. Insurers gain big in health reform's first year. *Market Watch*, March 22, 2011.
1.2 Ibid # 5.
13. Gentry, C. How much are you worth to HMOs? *Health News Florida*, October

28, 2011.

14. Dafny, L, Duggan, M, Ramanarayanan, S. Paying a premium on your premium? Consolidation in the U.S. health insurance industry. University of California at Los Angeles, 2010.

15. Schoen, C, Fryer, AK, Collins, SR, Radley, DC. State trends in premiums and deductibles, 2003-2010: The need for action to address rising costs. New York. The Commonwealth Fund, November 17, 2011.

16. Sorkin, AR. Huge buyout of hospital group highlights era of going private. *New York Times*, July 25, 2006: A1.

17. Zuckerman, G. A windfall for HCA investors. *Wall Street Journal*, March 4, 2011: C1.

18. Berenson, RA, Bazzoli, FGI, Au, M. Do specialty hospitals promote price competition? Center for Studying Health System Change. Issue Brief No. 103, January, 2006.

19. Mathews, AW. Hospitals put on sick list. *Wall Street Journal*, August 10, 2011.

20. Hsia, RY, Kellermann, AL, Shen, YC. Factors associated with closures of emergency departments in the United States. *JAMA*, May 18, 2011.

21. O'Malley, AS, Bond, AM. Berenson, RA. Rising hospital employment of physicians: better quality, higher costs? Center for Studying Health System Change. Issue Brief No. 136, August 2011.

22. Doyle, J. Outpatient sticker shock: $538 for a 3-minute treatment. *Post Dispatch*, November 27, 2011. (htpp://www.stltoday.com/business/local/outpatient-sticker-shock…)

23. Harrington, C, Hauser, C, Olney, B, Rosenau, PV. Ownership, financing, and management strategies of the ten largest for-profit nursing home chains in the United States. *Intl J Health Services* 41 (4): 725-46, 2011.

24. Harrington, C, Olney, B, Carrillo, H, Kang, T. Nurse staffing and deficiencies in the largest for-profit nursing home chains and chains owned by private equity companies. *Health Services Research* 47 (1): 106-28, 2012.

25. Mathews, AW, Rockoff, JD. Megadeal unites drug rivals. *Wall Street Journal*, July 22, 2011: B1.

26. Mathews, AW. Deal, combining two big rivals, will attract scrutiny. *Wall Street Journal*, July 22, 2011: B2.

27. Martin, GW. Walgreen prescribes a rate change. *Wall Street Journal*, October 25. 2011: B1.

28. Colliver, V, Pender, K. Walgreens spat sends millions to new pharmacies. *SFGate.com*, January 12, 2012.

29. Ibid # 10.

30. Austin, DA, Hungerford, TL. *The Market Structure of the Health Insurance Industry*. Washington, D.C. Congressional Research Service, November 17, 2009.

31. Gold, J. ACO is the hottest three-letter word in health care. *Kaiser Health News*, October 21, 2011.

32. Woolhandler, S, Himmelstein, DU. ACOs: a brief comment on an untested theory. Chicago, IL. *PNHP Newletter*. Fall 2011, p 54.

The Promise:
FREE MARKETS SPUR EFFICIENCY

CHAPTER 6

Trading Efficiency For Profits: How Bureacracy And Waste Are Multiplied, Not Reduced, In Private Health Care

Market theorists and proponents have told us for so many years that the private competitive marketplace in health care is more efficient than any publicly financed program. Many now accept this claim as the "American way" without questioning its basis in fact. This is part of the political rationale that has been used to justify all system "reform" efforts over the past 30 years.

It is long overdue to seriously question this premise. As the last two chapters have shown, the deregulated private marketplace in health care is filled with perverse incentives to raise revenues, costs and prices, all to the benefit of stakeholders on the supply side. How accurate are the market claims of higher efficiency and less bureaucracy compared to publicly financed health care?

This chapter takes on three goals: (1) to compare market rhetoric with reality and track record in terms of efficiency and bureaucracy; (2) to discuss how market efficiency is an unattainable goal within a profit-driven health care system dependent on fee-for-service (FFS) reimbursement; and (3) to briefly consider various types of efficiency and how they relate to the kind of health care we would like to have.

MARKETS: RHETORIC VS. REALITY

Among the many claims by neoconservative economist of the alleged increased efficiency of the private health care marketplace, publications by John Goodman, health economist at the Dallas-based National Center for Policy Analysis (NCPA), stand out as the most assertive, detailed—and wrong-headed. This well-funded right-wing think tank has been prolific in its reports over the years, including its extensive 2002 report, *Twenty Myths about Single-Payer Health Insurance: International Evidence on the Effects of National Health Insurance in Countries Around the World.* While acknowledging that other advanced countries contain costs better than we do in this country, the report claims that they do so by denying services, not by using resources more efficiently. It further asserts that our shorter hospital stays are evidence of more efficiency, touting the actuarial and consulting firm Milliman & Robertson as the "market leader in devising [managed care] guidelines" for more "efficient" practice. Concerning health insurance, the report goes on to say:

> "Single-payer health insurance differs from many private insurance companies in one important respect—no profit motive. But, far from [stockholders] being a burden, having no stockholders removes any incentive to operate efficiently. In fact, national health insurance provides all the wrong incentives for both the health care system itself and the patients in the system." [1]

The many claims of the NCPA report have been rebutted in detail elsewhere.[2] Concerning claims of greater market efficiencies with less bureaucracy, we have all kinds of evidence to the contrary:

- As a single-payer program serving the elderly for more than four decades, Medicare operates with administrative overhead of no more than 3 percent; private health insurers are five to nine times more expensive.[3]
- Despite their higher overhead, private insurers also have much higher error rates. Medicare has an error rate for claims processing of 4 percent. In contrast, a 2011 report by the AMA found that private payers have an average claims-processing error rate of 19.3 percent. Anthem Blue Cross/Blue Shield, a poster child for

private health insurance, had an error rate of 39 percent in 2010! Moreover, the AMA report found that physicians received no payment at all on almost 23 percent of claims they submitted to private insurers.[4]

- With some 1,300 private insurers in the U.S., fragmentation, inefficiency, and duplicative bureaucracy are the rule for insurers, and a frustrating reality for providers and patients alike. According to Dr. Allan Korn, medical director of the Chicago-based Blue Cross Blue Shield Association, Chicago has about 17,000 different insurance plan designs;[5] in another study of 2,000 patients with depression in Seattle, they were covered by 189 different plans with 755 different policies.[6]
- Between 2000 and 2005, while the insurance market declined by 1 percent, its workforce grew by one-third.[7]
- The Milliman & Robertson guidelines for efficient managed care have been considered medically unsafe by many physicians; as one example, one such guideline recommended hospital stays of only three days for *complicated* appendectomy, while a national study of 2,400 U.S. hospitals found average lengths of stay for such patients of 5.3 days.[8]

What is the rebuttal by proponents of our private financing system to these glaring inefficiencies? One example of private multi-payer financing is the Massachusetts health reform effort, initiated in 2006 and touted by some as a model for U.S. reform. In terms of efficiency and cost containment, it is already a failure. While Massachusetts has achieved near-universal coverage through a variety of complex mechanisms, it is now saddled with increased costs, more inefficiency and growing bureaucracy. Over its initial three-year period, health care employment in administrative jobs per capita grew by 18.4 percent compared to a national average of 8 percent.[9]

One implication of all this inefficiency is clear. More than 4,700 U.S. physicians responded to Medscape's 2011 Insurer Ratings Report with vitriolic anger over private insurers' unjustified denial of claims, needless pre-authorization demands, and requests for further documentation that are perceived as ways to stall payment as long as possible.[10]

Comparisons with our neighbor to the north convincingly counter any claims of increased efficiency and less bureaucracy in our supposedly competitive market-based system. Consider these two:

- A 2003 study measured how many administrative employees there are for every 10,000 enrollees of U.S. private insurers, and compared that number with administrative staff required for two provinces in Canada. The differences are striking, as shown in Figure 6.1.[11]
- A 2011 study compared how much U.S. physician practices spend per physician per year relating to payers compared to their counterparts in Canada's single-payer system. The result: U.S. physicians spend nearly four times the amount of money per physician per year relating to payers than their counterparts in Ontario, Canada ($82,975 vs. $22,205). U.S. nursing staff spends 20.6 hours per physician per week interacting with health plans, almost ten times that spent by Canadian nurses in dealing with their single-payer system. Much of that time is consumed in dealing with differences among insurers in drug formularies (which can change frequently); the specifics of contracts with laboratories, hospitals, specialists and drug companies; and seeking prior authorization for planned tests or consultations.[12] Table 6.1 shows these differences for two major areas—claims/billing and prior authorizations.[13]

Other parts on the supplier side of the medical-industrial-complex have their own administrative bureaucracies, also increasing all the time as each stakeholder prepares to better position itself to adapt to whatever changes will come about as various provisions of the ACA are implemented in the next few years. Despite the continuing recession and bad economy, the health care sector turns out to be the country's top job generator. According to the Bureau of Labor Statistics, health care accounts for 20 percent of all new jobs created in the year 2010 to 2011. Of the 80,000 net new U.S. jobs in October 2011 alone, 12,000 were in health care, ranging from hospitals, physicians' offices, and clinics to laboratories, nursing homes and home health care agencies. Most of these are administrative, including administrators, clerks, billing specialists, and information technology workers. Some hospitals find themselves cutting clinical and nursing staff even as they add new administrative positions.[14]

FIGURE 6.1

Number of Administrative Employees per 10,000 Enrollees, Nine U.S. Health Insurance Companies and Two Provincial Health Insurance Plans

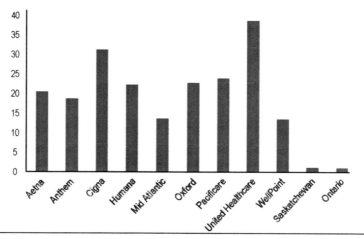

Source. Reprinted with permission from Woolhandler, S, Campbell, T, Himmel stein, DU. Costs of health care administration in the United States and Canada. *N Engl J Med* 349: 368, 2003.

TABLE 6.1

Mean Hours Per Physician Per Week Spent on Interactions With Payers in Canada and The United States

PERSONNEL	CLAIMS BILLING	PRIOR AUTHORIZATIONS
Canada		
Physicians	1.2	—
Nurses	1.2	—
Clerical Staff	15.9	—
Senior Administrators (hrs/year)	23.5	—
United States		
Physicians	0.9	1.0
Nurses	3.8	13.1
Clerical Staff	45.5	6.3
Senior Administrators (hrs/year)	173.7	.03

Source: Morra, D, Nicholson, S, Levinson, W, Gans, DN, Hammons, T et al. U.S. physician practices versus Canadians: spending nearly four times as much money interacting with payers. *Health Affairs* 30 (8): 1443-50, 2011.

For those believing that the present multi-payer "competitive" marketplace is more efficient and less bureaucratic than publicly financed programs, the Community Tracking Study (CTS) conducted by the non-profit Center for Studying Health System Change (HSC) may be enlightening. Since 1996, it has conducted site visits every two years tracking change in 12 randomly selected, nationally representative metropolitan communities (Boston, Cleveland, Greenville, SC, Indianapolis, Lansing, Little Rock, Miami, northern New Jersey, Orange County, CA, Phoenix, Seattle, and Syracuse, NY). Its 2004 report was based on periodic interviews in sixty communities with 60,000 households and 12,000 physicians, together with additional surveys of employers and insurers. Over the first seven years of the study, almost 2,700 interviews were completed.

In that report, the CTS identified these four major barriers to efficient health systems in the communities studied:

- Providers had enough market power in most sites to set their own prices, dictate the terms of their arrangements with health plans, and sidestep pressures to provide technically efficient care.
- Most physician markets were so fragmented that the potential efficiencies of integrated delivery systems were not achievable.
- Employers lacked the clout to push the their local systems toward efficiency and quality.
- There was insufficient health plan competition to engender more efficient local health care systems.[15]

The CTS drew this overall conclusion after seven years of study, rebutting the theory that markets produce efficiency: "Based on repeated site visits to the same twelve communities, the path to a more efficient health care system is blocked by a lack of effective competition among providers."[16]

MARKET EFFICIENCY: AN UNATTAINABLE GOAL IN A MULTI-PAYER, FEE-FOR-SERVICE DRIVEN SYSTEM

In separating rhetoric and wishful thinking by market theorists from the actual track record of how these theories play out in health care, the forgoing shows that widespread inefficiencies and increasing bureaucracy continue to plague our profit-driven market-based system. All reform attempts by Congress over the last 30-plus years have attempted to build on the "strengths" of private deregulated health care markets, with all leading to the same unachievable results in terms of cost containment, greater efficiency and value of care.

To be fair, we have to recognize that free market competition may work fine in many other sectors of the economy in giving customers lower prices, more choice, and better value. But as we have said in earlier chapters, health care is very different from buying a car or other goods where information can often be more transparent, where competitors compete by price and service, where time for decision-making is often less urgent, and where consumers have more clout than do patients. People covered by employer-sponsored health insurance find themselves limited by decisions made by their employer and insurer. Other kinds of insurance also limit their choices, all of which are strongly influenced by ability to pay. Especially in acute care situations, patients' options are restricted to physicians and facilities that are available to them in their own community. And as we have described in the forgoing, competition among providers on the supply side of our health care marketplace does *not* result in lower prices or better value.

So we still have to ask whether the free market approach in health care can *ever* be successful in gaining efficiencies still promoted by laissez faire theorists. Here I propose that we will *never* get to an efficient health care system that is affordable, sustainable, and meets the needs of our population for necessary health care by following the directions urged by free market advocates. Three big and interacting barriers stand in the way:

- *The multi-payer insurance industry itself.* Its products are *more* administrative products and costs. Most of the industry chases profits over service through many successful strategies that select healthier enrollees, and avoid coverage of sicker patients. As the watered-down ACA comes closer to implementation of (slightly) more rigorous requirements for medical-loss ratios (MLRs), insurers keep trying to label some of their administrative costs as "patient care"; request (and get) federal waivers of other requirements; and work their ways around firm rate-setting of their premiums. Much of their administrative overhead still involves denial management and marketing of underinsurance products. With some 1,300 competing private insurers, their collective administrative costs represent waste (and potential savings) as high as $380 billion a year, according to calculations comparing the 31 percent administrative health care costs in this country with those in Canada's single-payer system.[17,18]

- *Fee-for-service payment system and payment "reforms" now being considered.* We have already seen that almost all of organized medicine, whether the AMA or many specialty societies, fights against any threats to its present revenue. FFS gives many physicians a chance to offset reimbursement cuts by increasing the volume of services. Billing codes are an administrative nightmare, with the government a contributing player as long as we have a FFS payment system. The *10th Revision of the International Classification of Diseases*, scheduled to come on line in 2013, expands the number of billing codes from 18,000 to 140,000 (not a typo!). Examples defy logic or reason; these new codes illustrate: W22.02XA ("walked into a lamppost, initial encounter"), and V91.07XA ("burn due to water-skis on fire"); what has been a single billing code for a badly healed fracture could now generate 2,595 different codes! Needless to say, this change will add greatly to physicians' administrative overhead costs while adding many new jobs for billing clerks and consulting companies.[19] The ACA does call for development of new billing methods, such as encouraging integrated care through "bundled payments." But after three years of an initial "road test" of the PROMETHEUS bundled payment model, pilot participants had not by 2011 been able to make bundled payments or execute new payment contracts. Another theory may well bite the dust. PROMETHEUS (an acronym for *Provider Payment Reform for Outcomes, Margins, Evidence, Transparency, Hassle Reduction, Excellence, Understandability, and Sustainability)* is intended to lump together payment for all of the care needed for defined clinical episodes, such as acute myocardial infarction and hip replacement. This initiative, however, turns out to be extremely complex.

  Although three pilot sites are using electronic medical

records (EMRs), they still lack capabilities to make the redesign more effective. Even as this "reform" tries to get off the ground, bureaucracy has further increased, no cost savings have been generated, and physicians can be expected to oppose such a system if it limits their incomes.[20]

- *Lack of adequate regulation.* Although we hear ongoing pushback from the right and corporate stakeholders about "over-regulation" of our health care system, we continue to have a largely deregulated, laissez faire system. As examples, insurers have many ways to get around regulations in many states[21], the Obama administration has waived many of the initial requirements of the ACA[22], and the drug industry has fended off price controls for all these years.

The latest iteration of the aforementioned CTS hammers in even more nails in the coffin of efficiency through market forces. In its 2011 report, based on 2010 site visits, the study found lingering fallout of the ongoing recession, with slowing of the demand for health care (especially for elective procedures), and increased costs without greater efficiencies.[23]

WHAT IS EFFICIENCY ANYWAY?

This is a more complicated question than most of us realize, especially market theorists who see efficiency as the most streamlined way to extract profits form the health care market. We are indebted to Marc Roberts, professor of political economy and health policy at the Harvard School of Public Health, for expanding our definitions of "efficiency." As he points out: "to be efficient means to use our resources in the best possible way to achieve our ends." But that means that the definition of efficiency depends on what our goals in health care are.[24]

If we look at how our present system is constructed and actually works, as described in earlier chapters, we have to conclude that it is largely a profit-oriented venture within an enormous, minimally regulated medical-industrial-complex. It is based on ability to pay, not medical need, with wide gaps in income across our population defining the level of care received. Compared to other advanced countries around the world, we are "exceptional" in not yet having answered, as a society, these kinds of fundamental questions concerning our health care goals: who is the health care system for—patients and families or corporate stakeholders on the supply side?; should it be for-profit or not-for-profit?; is health care a right, or just a commodity for sale on an open market?; and is there a role for government in assuring that all Americans get necessary care?

Marc Roberts defines "efficiency" in four very different ways as related to goals:

- a *needs* approach which maximizes the overall or average health of a target population.
- a *demand* approach that gives people what they want if they can afford it (e.g. consumer-directed health care), but does not accommodate those who can't pay.
- *distributive efficiency*, whereby gains in health care are well distributed throughout the population on an equitable basis.
- *dynamic efficiency*, which focuses on finding new ways to treat patients that *reduce* the costs of care instead of increasing costs, as so many of today's innovations do. In this respect, Roberts has this to say: [To attain distributive efficiency] "we need to move from fee-for-service payment (which often encourages the overuse of expensive new drugs and procedures) to bundled payments for episodes of illness or capitated payments that cover all of a given person's costs for the year. Only then will hospitals and doctors find that efficiency—which research shows, ironically, also often produces better clinical outcomes—is in their interest. And only then will entrepreneurs and scientists have an incentive to develop those cost-reducing innovations, thereby really increasing our efficiency where it counts."[25]

Unfortunately, the level of debate over the kind of health care that we want continues to avoid the fundamental questions that we will need to resolve if we are to achieve real health care reform that is sustainable. At this point, this observation by Jamie Court, president of Consumer Watchdog and author of *The Progressive's Guide to Raising Hell*, tells it how it is:

"There's no denying that the United States has the most costly and least efficient system in the world. Every other national health care system in the world has someone watching the money and a national discussion of how it should reasonably be spent. In America, employers pay health insurers to say 'no', because they don't want to have to. When Congress started to discuss the issue of what's reasonable to pay for and not to pay for at the end of life, the cash-rich opponents of change effectively raised the specter of 'death panels.'" [26]

In sum, we have to conclude that conservatives' long-held view that health care markets are more efficient than more regulated markets is blatant disinformation defying the evidence. We have to see it for what it is—self-serving rhetoric of stakeholders determined to perpetuate the status quo. But they also tell us that markets will somehow bring us better quality of care. We'll consider that claim in the next chapter.

References

1. Goodman, JC, Herrick, DM. Twenty Myths about Single-Payer Health Insurance: International Evidence on the Effects of National Health Insurance in Countries Around the World. National Center for Policy Analysis, Dallas, 2002, pp 38, 64.
2. Geyman, JP. Myths and memes about single-payer health insurance in the United States: a rebuttal to conservative claims. *Intl J Health Services 35 (1): 63-90, 2005.*
3. Woolhandler, S, Himmelstein, DU. The National Health Program Slide-Show Guide, Center for National Health Program Studies, Cambridge, MA, 2000.
4. AMA. New AMA health insurer report card finds increasing inaccuracy in claims payment. American Medical Association, June 20, 2011.
5. Kagel, R. Blue crossroads: Insurance in the 21st Century. *American Medical News*, September 20, 2004.
6. Grembowski, DE, Diehr, P, Novak, LC, Roussel, AF, Morton, DP. Measuring the "managedness" and covered benefits of health plans. *Health Services Research* 35 (3): 707, 2000.
7. Krugman, P. The world of U.S. health care economics is downright scary. *Seattle Post Intelligencer*, September 26, 2006: B1.
8. Martinez, B. Care guidelines used by insurers face scrutiny. *Wall Street Journal, September 14, 2000.*
9. Staiger, DO, Auerbach, DI, Buerhaus, PI. Health care reform and the health care workforce—the Massachusetts experience. *N Engl J Med* 365 (12): e24, September 7, 2011.

10. Kaiser Health News. Survey finds physicians unhappy with insurance companies. December 6, 2011.
11. Woolhandler, S, Costs of health care administration in the United States and Canada. *N Engl J Med* 349 (): 768-75, 2003.
12. Chen, PW. Many health plans, many hours spent haggling. *New York Times,* August 30, 2011: D5.
13. Morra, D, Nicholson, S, Levinson, W, Gans, DN, Hammons, T et al. U.S. physician practices versus Canadians: spending nearly four times as much money interacting with payers. *Health Affairs* 30 (8): 1443-50, 2011.
14. Mitchell, R. Hospitals gear hiring to health law and industry changes. *Kaiser Health News,* November 30, 2011.
15. Nichols, LM, Ginsburg, PB, Berenson, RA, Christianson, J, Hurley, RE. Are market forces strong enough to deliver efficient health care systems? Confidence is waning. *Health Affairs* 23 (2): 8-21, 2004.
16. Ibid # 14, p. 17.
17. Ibid # 10.
18. Woolhandler, S. Cutting costs by reducing the bureaucracy. Letter to the Editor. *New York Times,* November 20, 2011.
19. Mathews, AW. Walked into a lamppost? Hurt while crocheting? Help is on the way. *Wall Street Journal,* September 13, 2011: A1.
20. Hussey, PS. Ridgely, MS, Rosenthal, MB. The PROMETHEUS bundled payment experiment: slow start shows problems in implementing new payment models. *Health Affairs* 30 (11): 2116-24, 2011.
21. Geyman, JP. *Do Not Resuscitate: Why the Health Insurance Industry is Dying, and How We Must Replace It.* Monroe, ME. Common Courage Press, 2008, pp. 105-7.
22. Geyman, JP. Waiving away affordability of health care. *Huffington Post,* December 9, 2010.
23. Felland, LE, Grossman, Tu, HT. Key findings from HSC's 2010 site visits. Health care markets weather economic downturn, brace for health reform. Issue Brief No. 135. Washington, D.C. Center for Studying Health System Change, May 2011.
24. Roberts, MJ. Efficiency: getting clear on our goals. Connecting American Values with Health Reform. The Hastings Center, September 30, 2009.
25. Ibid # 23.
26. Court, J. *The Progressive's Guide to Raising Hell: How to Win Grassroots Campaigns, Pass Ballot Box Laws, and Get the Change We Voted For.* White River Junction, VT. Chelsea Green Publishing, 2010, p. 97.

The Promise:
HEALTH CARE MARKETS BOOST QUALITY OF CARE

CHAPTER 7

Markets Bring Us the Best Health Care in the World—Right?

Having looked in the last chapter at the argument that we need free markets to create efficiency in health care, we turn to another argument: competition spurs quality.

In some sectors, such as the computer industry, we have seen rapid increases in quality under heavy competition among businesses driven to distinguish themselves from their rivals.

But, as we saw in the last chapter, competition in the health care industry leads to *decreased* efficiency. What about quality? Does our market-based system deliver better health care, for both individuals and our population, even if it is inefficient and costs much more than in other advanced countries?

Many people believe, or take for granted, that we have the best health care in the world here in America. This view is fueled by conservative think tanks and corporate stakeholders in our market-based system as part of a conservative mantra holding that competitive markets will assure better access to more affordable care of better quality. As an example, the 2002 report from the National Center for Policy Analysis mentioned in an earlier chapter, *Twenty Myths about Single-Payer Health Insurance: International Evidence on the Effects of National Health Insurance in Countries around the World,* touted this country's greater access and use of medical technology as a rationale for this view while discrediting the validity of such outcome measures as life expectancy and mortality rates in international comparisons. The report bypassed a rich literature of cross-national studies on the quality of health care, asserting that such factors as race, income or geography have little to do with quality. While acknowledging that we pay more for health care than other countries, the report held that "we also get more and what we get may save lives." [1]

This chapter has three goals: (1) to discuss various definitions of quality of health care, and how it is measured; (2) to examine the track record of health care markets in terms of quality of care delivered; and (3) to briefly consider what lessons we can learn from this track record in terms of health policy going forward.

WHAT IS QUALITY AND HOW IS IT MEASURED?

At the outset, these may appear to be simple questions, but they are not. We have seen more progress on the definition side than on the measurement side. But despite all of our technological progress, even the definition of quality is a work in progress.

We are indebted to the Institute of Medicine (IOM) for this 1990 definition of "quality": "the degree to which health services for individuals and populations increase the likelihood of desired health outcomes and are consistent with current professional knowledge." [2] In an important 1998 article, Schuster and his colleagues added: "good quality means providing patients with appropriate services in a technically competent manner, with good communication, shared decision making, and cultural sensitivity." [3] Three years later, in its landmark 2001 report *Crossing the Quality Chasm: A New Health System for the 21st Century,* the Institute of Medicine identified these six key dimensions of quality of health care: [4]

1. *Safe*—avoiding injuries to patients from the care that is intended to help them.
2. *Effective*—providing services based on scientific knowledge to all who could benefit and refraining from providing services to those not like to benefit (avoiding underuse and overuse, respectively).
3. *Patient-centered*—providing care that is respectful of and responsive to individual patient preferences, needs, and values and ensuring that patient values guide all clinical decisions.
4. *Timely*—reducing waits and sometimes harmful delays for both those who receive and those who give care.

5. *Efficient*—avoiding waste, including waste of equipment, supplies, ideas, and energy.
6. *Equitable*—providing care that does not vary in quality because of personal characteristics such as gender, ethnicity, geographic location, and socioeconomic status."[4]

As we have already seen in earlier chapters, access, costs, and affordability of health care are intertwined such that there can be *no* quality of care without access to essential services. In its concerns over barriers to access that lead to disparities in the quality of care received by patients with cancer, the American Cancer Society launched a national effort in 2007 calling for "4 A's coverage":

- *Adequate*—timely access to the full range of evidence-based health care including prevention and early detection.
- *Affordable*—costs are based on the person's ability to pay.
- *Available*—coverage available regardless of health status or prior claims.
- *Administratively simple*—processes are easy to understand and navigate.[5]

That formulation is especially relevant since the single most important aspect of access to care for patients with cancer is the status of their insurance coverage.[6]

There are many subtleties that influence how useful any of these definitions are when it comes to quality of care. For instance, inappropriate or unnecessary care is of poor quality even if provided in a technically competent way. Health outcomes that are intermediate, such as improvements in laboratory tests, often have nothing to do with outcomes that matter to patients, such as quality of life, morbidity or mortality.

Measurement of health care quality is even more challenging than its definition. There are three basic categories of measures—*structure* (such as characteristics of physicians and hospitals), *process* (that involve providers and their patients), and *outcomes* (relating to the patient's subsequent health status).[7] Most of the quality assurance measures used by insurers and managed care organizations are *process* measures that may have little to do with improved outcomes. Dr. Tom

Bodenheimer, co-director of the Center for Excellence in Primary Care at the University of California, San Francisco, gives us this observation concerning the difficulties in measuring quality of care:[8]

> "Each intervention requires its own particular measurements of quality; some elucidate the processes of care, and some focus on outcomes. . . . For patients with coronary artery disease, measures might include the percentage receiving aspirin and beta-blockers (process) and the percentage who have myocardial infarction or sudden death from cardiac causes (outcomes). Even when considering only one health care intervention—for example, coronary artery bypass surgery—it is treacherous to compare the outcomes of one surgical team with those of another without adjusting for the age of the patients and the severity of their illness."

Other difficulties in measuring quality of care include the unreliability of "report cards" for individual physicians, the ease with which high outlier physicians can game the system by pruning some of the sicker patients from their practice[9], and the challenge in measuring ambulatory care encounters, which often involve multiple clinical conditions.[10]

All this reminds me of a classic quote, repeated by others in various contexts, that applies to the multi-dimensional challenge of measuring quality of care—that what's the easiest to count doesn't much count, and that what really counts is hard (or impossible) to count.

MARKETS AND QUALITY: A DISCONNECT

There can be no denial that many Americans, especially if well insured and affluent, can gain access to the most advanced and best care in the world. But in contrast to what is available to some, access to affordable quality care is more than problematic for a large and growing part of our population, as is well documented by many studies here and by a large number of cross-national studies over many years. Our profit-driven market-based system exacerbates prevailing quality deficiencies and stands in the way of improvement.

Dr. Don Berwick, founder and former president and CEO of the

Institute for Healthcare Improvement, Harvard professor of pediatrics and health policy, and until recently head of the Centers for Medicare and Medicaid Services (CMS), recognized early on that *system change* will be required to achieve significant improvement in the quality of American health care. He argued that assuring quality in health care was not just a matter of identifying and removing a few bad apples, but instead requires a commitment to *continuous quality improvement* throughout our health care system. He has been a strong proponent of evidence-based medicine, and has been realistic in assessing the barriers to change within the system, be they physicians, other providers, hospitals, or other institutions. In a landmark 2003 article, he and his colleagues identified two main barriers to the use of information to motivate change:

> "*Pathway I* (selection), the lack of skill, knowledge, and motivation on the part of those who could drive change by using data to choose from among competing providers; and *Pathway II*, (change in health care delivery), the deficiencies in organizational and professional capacity in health care to lead change and improvement itself."[11]

Five Reasons for Poor and Unacceptable Quality in Our Market-Based System

Rather than enhancing quality of care throughout our system under the theory of market competition, market-based care instead does the opposite on a widespread and systemic basis for these five basic reasons. (Some markers documenting this pattern in earlier chapters are repeated here for clarity.)

1. Underuse of necessary services among uninsured and underinsured patients. Because we have a system based on ability to pay, not primarily medical need, many patients delay or forgo care altogether, as illustrated by these markers:

- 50,000 Americans die every year in the U.S. (136 per day) for lack of health insurance.[12]
- Women age 40 to 64 without insurance are only half as likely to have had a mammogram with the last two years compared to their insured counterparts.[13]

- One in four uninsured cancer patients delay or forgo care because of cost.[14]
- Uninsured African-American women with breast cancer have a five-year survival rate of only 63 percent compared to 89 percent for Caucasian women.[15]
- Cancer patients are three times more likely than their insured counterparts to have not seen a health care professional in the last year, twice as likely to have no regular source of care, and five times more likely to use the emergency room for care.[16]
- Medicaid enrollees are more likely to have late-stage cancers when diagnosed, resulting in worse outcomes.[17]

2. Overuse of inappropriate and unnecessary services. As we have seen in earlier chapter, market incentives for many physicians, hospitals and other facilities drive increased volume of well-reimbursed services whether clinically beneficial or not, as illustrated by these common examples:

- Up to one-third of all health care services provided each year are either inappropriate or unnecessary, and some are actually harmful.[18]
- Despite the lack of evidence of benefit or approval by the FDA or the American College of Radiology, more than 30 million full-body CT scans are performed each year for screening purposes.[19]
- Dr. Peter Bach, oncologist at Sloan-Kettering Cancer Center and former senior advisor on health care quality at CMS, estimates that 30 to 40 percent of spending on cancer care is of marginal value.[20]
- A 2008 study by United Health found that the anti-anemia drug Procrit was being over-prescribed by oncologists—one-third of patients were not anemic at all.[21]

3. Profits trump quality of care. That the quest for profits by supply-siders in the medical-industrial-complex frequently trumps service to patients is shown by these kinds of examples:

- Investor-owned hospitals, HMOs, nursing homes, and mental health centers provide more expensive care that is of worse quality compared to their not-for-profit counterparts.[22]
- The more specialists in an area, the higher the costs and the lower

the quality.[23]
- The drug industry pursues a comprehensive strategic plan to maximize sales and profits with insufficient concern for the safety and benefits of their products, as described by Donald W. Light in his excellent book *The Risks of Prescription Drugs*. (Table 7.1)[24]
- In order to reduce costs and increase profits, many drug companies outsource manufacturing of their drugs to other countries, in many cases compromising the quality of their products.[25]
- Mortality rates for the nation's two largest for-profit dialysis chains are 19 to 24 percent higher than not-for-profit chains.[26]
- For-profit hospices offer fewer services and provide worse quality of care compared to their not-for-profit counterparts.[27]

TABLE 7.1

Strategies by Big Drug Industry to Maximize Sales and Profits

1. Medicalize worries, perceived risks, and îdiseasesî for which people will take drugs.
2. Quickly approve as many apparently safe drugs as possible, whether clinically superior or not, based on trials designed by companies to minimize evidence of harms and maximize evidence of benefits.
3. Use surrogate endpoints around which whole models of risk can be constructed to create new markets of need.
4. Commercialize professional judgment. Have sales reps be the principal source of information, education, and advice about prescribing. Have marketing departments fund educational courses and professional conference sessions.
5. Reward de facto proliferation of unapproved uses to maximize sales, fueled by DTCA (direct-to-consumer advertising) and paid physician educators. Mass market for all plausible uses.
6. Monitor adverse events primarily through passive, voluntary reporting by the companies that profit from selling the drugs.
7. Have an underfunded, understaffed safety division with few powers to investigate and withdraw problem drugs and to warn and protect the public.
8. Have experts with industry ties set prescribing guidelines that maximaize the number of patient-consumers.

Source: Light, DW. *The Risks of Prescription Drugs*. New York. Columbia University Press, 2010, p. 159.

4. Oversight and regulation remain lax. As a principal federal agency for oversight and regulation of U.S. health care, the FDA is seriously hampered in its mission by under-funding, insufficient authority, close ties to the very industries that it is regulating, and political interference. These examples illustrate the point:

- A 2008 study found that among 90 drugs approved by the FDA between 1998 and 2000, only 394 of 909 clinical trials were ever published in a peer-reviewed journal; only one in five clinical trials for cancer ever made it into a medical journal.[28]
- Without any clinical evidence that a 23 mg dose of the Alzheimer's drug Aricept is more effective than a 10 mg dose (and that efficacy is open to some question), the FDA has recently approved the larger dose even though patients have stopped taking the drug twice as often as the 10 mg dose due to adverse side effects. Public Citizen's Health Research Group has filed a petition to the FDA calling for the immediate withdrawal from the market of the 23 mg dose because of its harmful side effects.[29]
- After an expedited 510 (k) review process, J&J's Gynecare Prolift mesh received FDA approval several years ago as a less invasive treatment for pelvic organ prolapse. As is often the case with such accelerated approvals that proceed without clinical trials or demonstrated efficacy, significant problems have followed, including treatment failures and deaths. The IOM has recently called for the FDA to require more rigorous review of the approval process.[30]
- Another medical device, J&J's A.S.R., a metal artificial hip replacement, received expedited FDA review and approval without clinical trials. But the devices have had a high failure rate, many patients have been disabled by pain as the device sheds metal debris, and many have needed to be removed. The device was recalled by the company in 2010. Until its use declined sharply after that recall, the A.S.R. accounted for almost one-third of an estimated 250,000 hip replacements performed each year in the U.S.[31]
- In order to lower costs and avoid FDA regulatory requirements, many drug companies outsource clinical trials to other countries;

as an example, more than 13,000 Peruvians participated in clinical trials for U.S.-bound drugs without any pre-approval or inspection by the FDA; oversight and protections for human subjects are lax in participating countries, and the contracting company can simply bury results that they don't like.[32]

- Always under pressure from industry (and often from patient advocates), the FDA allowed expanded marketing of off-label cancer drugs in 2009 despite the lack of clinical evidence of their effectiveness.[33]

Other parts of our regulatory apparatus also fall short of assuring public safety in health care. As one example, the National Practitioner Data Bank was created in 1986 to provide oversight of physicians, and reveal trends in disciplinary actions and malpractice awards. It was intended to be a useful resource for state medical boards, hospitals and insurers. Yet a recent investigative report by the *Kansas City Star* analyzed thousands of records in the Data Bank, finding 21 physicians with at least 10 malpractice payments who had never been disciplined by state medical boards.[34] As another example, a recent study by HHS's Office of Inspector General found that only one in seven adverse events, some involving patients' deaths, are reported in U.S. hospitals. Moreover, only a few of those reported and investigated led to changes in policies or practices.[35]

5. Conflicts of interest (COIs) abound between industry, government and the delivery system. We discussed a range of COIs involving physicians and industry in Chapter 3 (pps. 58-59). But they are only the tip of the iceberg. There are many more involving other parties that relate to the profit-making engine of health care and to what health care legislation is enacted. These examples suggest the extent of these COIs:

- Senator Orrin Hatch (R-Utah) has championed the dietary supplement industry in Utah for many years. He authored a 1994 federal law that allows supplement companies to make general health claims about their products without review of their safety or effectiveness. He has received hundreds of thousands of dollars in campaign contributions from the industry over the years, and has successfully fended off regulation of supplements on a number of occasions, despite the mounting evidence of the hazards of some (e.g. supplements spiked with steroids or other unapproved drugs, and even deaths from "natural" sleep remedies).[36]

- In response to high failure rates of kidney transplants at the University Medical Center in Las Vegas, Nevada that included several deaths, CMS moved to shut down the program. But after strong protests led by Representative Shelley Berkley (D-NV), CMS reversed its decision, coming to an agreement to keep the facility open under the management of her physician husband. He is a nephrologist now directing the program who also has joint ownership of 10 other dialysis centers in Nevada with DaVita, a major provider of kidney care in the U.S with more than 1,700 dialysis facilities. The successful turnaround of CMS policy was facilitated by campaign contributions to Rep. Berkley from Amgen (a major supplier of drugs to dialysis centers), as well as trade groups representing dialysis centers and nephrologists. The COI involved not only Rep. Berkley and her husband, Dr. Larry Lehrner, who ended up with a $738,000 annual contract with the hospital. These COIs were not mentioned or dealt with in negotiations with CMS.[37]

- Senator Max Baucus (D-MT), as chairman of the Senate Finance Committee in the run-up to the 2010 ACA, played a pivotal role in developing the final legislation. He actively kept single-payer off the table, even to the point of having eight activists in the Senate chambers arrested and handcuffed, then jailed overnight. His committee was instrumental in killing the public option. His COIs were obvious—having received $1,170,313 over his career from the insurance sector and $2,797,381 from the health sector, according to the Center for Responsive Politics.[38] In addition, Elizabeth Fowler, former vice president of public policy for WellPoint, was his chief health advisor and widely seen as the main architect of the final legislation. The mainstream media never reported her close ties to industry.[39]

- An early provision of the Senate health reform bill in 2009 would have placed a 5 percent tax on elective cosmetic surgery. It was immediately dubbed the "Botax" after the anti-wrinkle product Botox. The American Academy of Cosmetic Surgery launched a firestorm of protest, calling it a tax against women and the baby boomer generation,[40] and the AMA spoke out against the tax as the first federal levy against a medical procedure.[41] The proposed tax was quickly dropped from the bill.

- A 2007 study looked at conflicts of interest among authors of 56 cancer research articles published medical journals. Of those reports disclosing funding by industry, 84 percent were favorable to the product studied, compared to just 54 percent of reports without industry funding. Moreover, industry-funded research was much more likely to have no comparison arm (66 percent vs. 33 percent).[42]

WHAT LESSONS CAN WE DRAW FROM THE MARKETS' CLAIMS OF QUALITY?

Admittedly, there are many physicians, other health care professionals, and institutions within our health care system that deliver care of high quality. For the most part, they are not-for-profit and more integrated systems, with physicians often paid by salary instead of FFS. Examples include Group Health Cooperative of Puget Sound, the Mayo Clinic, and the Geisinger Health System in Pennsylvania. In some places, such as Grand Junction, Colorado, physicians and hospitals have cooperated in developing a high-quality, fully accessible regional system of care.[43]

There have also been many important efforts toward improving quality of U.S. health care over the years by dedicated professionals and concerned organizations. Especially noteworthy are the initiatives by the IOM, the Institute for Health Care Improvement, and the Agency for Health Care Policy and Research (AHCPR) (now the Agency for Healthcare Research and Quality, AHRQ). But all of these have fallen short of the mark, since they have not changed the system-wide FFS-driven quest for profits.

Most of our health care system is still dominated by a business "ethic" tied to maximal profits at the expense of service and quality of care, as we have seen in the forgoing. This is unsustainable and unacceptable. Based on the well-documented track record of this large part of the overall system, we are forced to draw these 12 conclusions:

1. *Deregulated markets in health care, contrary to the claims of theorists and advocates, do not place a high priority on quality of care—profits trump service and quality.*

   The present lack of accountability for quality of care is unacceptable. Unfettered health care markets have had their day—concerning quality, they have failed to deliver over some 30 years. The experiment is over. As Donald Berwick notes: "Health care is broken. The delivery system isn't working. That's the problem. We set up a delivery system which is fragmented, unsafe, not sufficiently patient-centered, full of waste, unreliable, despite . . . great efforts of the workforce. We built it wrong. It isn't built for modern times."[44]

2. *More oversight and regulation by government will be required for the private sector to improve the quality of care and operate in the public interest.*

   We will need a larger role for government at both federal and state levels to reset and assure that higher standards for quality are met by providers and institutions on the delivery side of health care services.

3. *Conflicts of interest are widespread, work against quality of care, and must be brought under control.*

   COIs are rarely disclosed, but even when they are, that doesn't fix the problem. We need to set higher ethical standards throughout the system, and apply sanctions where and when necessary.

4. *We need to get politics out of health care.*

   There is a science to clinical medicine as well as to health policy. We must achieve what the free market ideologists agree we need—efficiency, lower costs, and the best possible value in our health care. Blind ideology disconnected from evidence and experience has played too large a role for too long.

5. *We need to see health care for what it is—a basic human need, not just another commodity for sale on an open market.*

Other advanced countries have recognized this fundamental point for many years—we are the outlier in the world. We need to acknowledge that today's health care is not on an open market and never can be without a larger role of government to rein in market excesses. Few patients have the resources to cover what they need when they need it. Most patients are captive to forces that prevent the collective power of their pocketbooks to drive down prices and raise quality.

6. *Physicians and their organizations need to play a larger role in leading toward a better patient-centered health care system.*

The physician workforce increasingly is subservient to their employers and corporate masters. And most of organized medicine, including the AMA and most specialty societies, are more interested in reimbursement policies that affect them than those policies that will make care more accessible and of better quality for all Americans. This leaves a vacuum in clinical leadership. Insurers and hospitals don't provide care, except through the physicians and other health professionals whom they recruit or hire. Physicians can best guide health policy through objective and responsible evidence-based medicine.

Concerning the pressing need for universal coverage and real health care reform, could we ever imagine the AMA leaving its reactionary stance and taking a progressive view reform in the public interest? Actually, we might, based on this resolution by the AMA's social insurance committee in 1917, only 95 years ago:

> "The time is present when the profession should study earnestly to solve the questions of medical care that will arise under various forms of social insurance. Blind opposition, indignant repudiation, bitter denunciation of these laws is worse than useless: it leads nowhere and it leaves the profession in a position of helplessness as the rising tide of social development sweeps over it."[45]

That resolution was quickly killed in 1917 when the issue was further debated at the state level, so we shouldn't hold our breaths awaiting AMA action!

7. *In order to improve the quality of care and outcomes for our entire population, we will have to achieve a system of universal coverage.*

Health disparities are increasing as the gaps between the poor and the affluent widen further and as the middle class hollows out. For 50 million uninsured and the rapidly growing numbers of underinsured, even basic and necessary care is becoming out of reach. We cannot limit quality assurance to the needs of individual patients, but must also deal with outcomes for our population as a whole.

8. *We need to rebalance the distribution of specialties within the physician workforce to address the shortage of primary care specialties, geriatrics and psychiatry.*

Fragmentation within our specialist-dominated physician workforce compromises coordination and integration of care—especially for patients with multiple chronic conditions—thereby reducing quality of care.

As a 2010 report by the Josiah Macy Jr. Foundation on the present and future of primary care observed:

"Too often, patients with complex acute or chronic health conditions receive services from multiple health providers in multiple care settings that do not coordinate and communicate with each other. This is especially true for the vulnerable elderly and disabled populations. This lack of coordination and integration leads to a fragmented healthcare system in which patients experience questionable care with more errors, more waste and duplication, and little accountability for quality and cost efficiency."[46]

9. *We need better measures of quality of care than we now have, including outcomes that most matter to patients (e.g. quality of life).*

This will be an ongoing challenge—to move beyond process measures to a greater emphasis on outcomes for both individual patients and populations.

10. *The ACA cannot be counted on to fix our quality, cost or access system problems.*

This point has been made in detail in my 2010 book *Hijacked: The Road to Single Payer in the Aftermath of Stolen Health Care Reform*.[47] We can anticipate that insurers will continue to game the system in many of their usual ways, even inventing new ways, such as withholding risk management and health status data from regulators.[48] We can also expect physicians and hospitals to upcode their services and game ACOs and new payment systems to their own advantage.

11. *If we can apply evidence-based medicine more broadly, we can cut costs while improving quality of care by reducing inappropriate and unnecessary services.*

As we recall from earlier chapters, up to one-third of all health care services provided in our market-based system are either inappropriate or unnecessary, some even harmful. So reining in this expensive waste and excess would obviously save large amounts of money while improving quality of care.

12. *We must work to improve the quality of U.S health care, both for individuals and for our population.*

We cannot be complacent about quality deficiencies in our market-based system. Our system is neither unique nor exceptional by world standards. It is inferior in quality to that of many advanced countries. As we saw earlier in Chapter 2 (pps 37-39), we have a long way to go to catch up with performance outcomes in many other advanced countries.[49]

As the political battles are waged over health care reform during this election cycle and as implementation of ACA draws closer, we can expect frenzied pushback by the major players trying to protect their prerogatives and profits. Examples abound at this writing (April 2012), including hospitals merging and building expanded physician networks; insurers buying up physician groups or developing new risk-sharing relationships; some insurers partnering with hospitals; and physician groups trying to protect their clinical autonomy even as they become employed by either hospitals or insurers (by 2013 only one-third of the nation's physicians are expected to own their own practices).[50]

In Chapter 12, we will return to the question of how we might change course toward a safer, more equitable and accountable health care system with greater access and higher quality. But at this point, it is time to move to the next chapter, where we will ask whether private markets can give us reliability and security of our own health care.

References

1. Goodman, JC, Herrick, DM. *Twenty Myths about Single-Payer Health Insurance: International Evidence on the Effects of National Health Insurance in Countries around the World.* National Center for Policy Analysis. Dallas, 2002, p. 31.
2. Lohr, KN (ed). *Medicare: A Strategy for Quality Assurance.* Washington, D.C. National Academy Press, 1990.
3. Schuster, M, McGlynn EA, Brook, RH. How good is the quality of health care in the United States? *Milbank Q.* 76(4): 517-63, 1998.
4. Institute of Medicine. Committee on Quality of Health Care in America. *Crossing the Quality Chasm: A New Health System for the 21st Century.* Washington, D.C. 2001.
5. Sack, K. Cancer society focuses its ads on the uninsured. *New York Times,* August 31, 2007.
6. Siminoff, LA, Ross, L. Access and equity to cancer care in the USA: a review and assessment. *Postgrad Med J* 81: 674, 2005.
7. Brook, RH, McGlynn, EA, Cleary, PD. Part 2: Measuring quality of care. *N Engl J Med* 335: 966-70, 1996.
8. Bodenheimer, T. The American health care system: The movement for improved quality in health care. *N Engl J Med* 340: 488-92, 1999.
9. Hofer, TP, Hayward, RA, Greenfield, S, Wagner, EH, Kaplan, SH et al. The unreliability of individual physician "report cards" for assessing the costs and quality of care of a chronic disease. *JAMA* 281: 2098-2105, 1999.
10. Fihn, SD. The quest to quantify quality. *JAMA* 283: 1740-42, 2000.
11. Berwick, DM, James, B, Coye, MJ. Connections between quality measurement and improvement. *Medical Care* 41 (1): I-30-I-38, 2003.
12. Wolfe, SM. Outrage of the Month! 50 million uninsured in the U.S. equals 50,000+ avoidable deaths each year. *Health Letter* 28 (1): 11, January 2012.
13. Ward, E, Halpern, M, Schrag, N et al. Association of insurance with cancer care utilization and outcomes. *CA Cancer J Clin* 58: 19-20, 2008.
14. Ibid # 12.
15. Bid # 12.
16. Wilper, AP, Woolhandler, S, Lasser, KE et al. A national study of chronic disease prevalence and access to care in uninsured U.S. adults. *Ann Intern Med* 149: 170-6, 2008.

17. Halpern, MT, Ward, EM, Pavluck, AL et al. Association of insurance status and ethnicity with cancer stage at diagnosis for 12 cancer sites: a retrospective analysis. *Lancet Oncol* 9 (3): 222-31, 2008.

18. Wenner, JB, Fisher, ES, Skinner, JS. Geography and the debate over Medicare reform. *Health Affairs Web Exclusive* W-103, February 13, 2002.

19. Brenner, DJ, Hall, EJ. Computed tomography—an increasing source of radiation exposure. *N Engl J Med* 357: 2277-84, 2007.

20. Bach, P., as quoted in McNeil, C. Sticker shock sharpens focus on biologics. News. *J Natl Cancer Inst* 99 (12): 911, 2007.

21. Culliton, BJ. Interview: Insurers and 'targeted biologics' for cancer: A conversation with Lee N. Newcomer. *Health Affairs Web Exclusive* 27 (1): W41-W51, 2008.

22. Geyman, JP. *The Corrosion of Medicine: Can the Profession Reclaim Its Moral Legacy?* Monroe, ME. Common Courage Press, 2008, p. 37.

23. Baicker, K, Chandra, A. Medicare spending, the physician workforce, and beneficiaries' quality of care. *Health Affairs (Millwood)* 23: w 184-9, 2004.

24. Light, DW. *The Risks of Prescription Drugs*. New York. Columbia University Press, 2010, p. 159.

25. Loftus, P. New lapses at J&J's Doxil supplier. *Wall Street Journal*, December 9, 2011: B4.

26. Zhang, Y, Cotter, DJ, Thamer, M. The effect of dialysis claims on mortality among patients receiving dialysis. *Health Services Research* 46 (3): 747-67, 2011.

27. Perry, J, Stone, R. In the business of dying: Questioning the commercialization of hospice. *Journal of Law, Medicine and Ethics*, May 18, 2011.

28. Hotz, RL. What you didn't know about a drug can hurt you: Untold numbers of clinical-trial results go unpublished; those that are made public can't always be believed. *Wall Street Journal*, December 12, 2008: A 16.

29. Holzer, B. FDA ignores negative feedback on Alzheimer's drug Aricept. *Public Citizen News* 31 (4): 20, 2011.

30. Wang, SS. FDA panel takes second look. *Wall Street Journal*, September 8, 2011: B6.

31. Meier, B. Metal hips failing fast, report says. *New York Times*, September 16, 2011: B1.

32. Hearn, K. The other South American drug war. U.S. regulators are turning a blind eye to the dramatic rise of clinical trials south of the border. *The Nation* 293 (15): 18-22, 2011.

33. Abelson, R, Pollack, A. Medicare widens drugs it accepts for cancer care: More off-label uses. *New York Times*, January 27, 2009.

34. Wilson, D. Withdrawal of database on doctors is protested. *New York Times*, September 16, 2011: B3.

35. Pear, R. Report finds most errors at hospitals unreported. *New York Times*, January 6, 2012: A12.

36. Lipton, E. Support is mutual for senator and makers of supplements. *New York Times*, June 21, 2011: A1.

37. Lipton, E. Nevada congresswoman's cause is often her husband's gain. *New*

York Times, September 6, 2011: A1.

38. Editorial. Puppets in Congress. *New York Times*, November 17, 2009: A28.

39. Connor, K. Chief health aide to Baucus is former WellPoint executive. *Eyes on the Ties* Blog, September 1, 2009.

40. Galewitz, P. Plastic surgeons cry foul over 'Botax' proposal in Senate health bill. *Kaiser Health News*, November 20, 2009.

41. Rockoff, JD. Knives drawn over 'Botax'. *Wall Street Journal*, December 4, 2009: A3.

42. Riechelmann, RP, Wang, L, O'Carroll, A et al. Disclosure of conflicts of interest by authors of clinical trials and editorials in oncology. *J Clin Oncol* 25 (29): 4642-47, 2007.

43. West, D, Mesa County, Colorado, health care: the best health care in the United States. Aurora: Colorado Academy of Family Physicians, August 2009. (htpp://www.coloradoafp.org)

44. Berwick, D. as quoted by Galewitz, P. Transcript: Donald Berwick on Medicare, Medicaid, 'rationing' and who decides. *Kaiser Health News*, December 12, 2011.

45. Burrow, JG. *AMA: Voice of American Medicine*. Baltimore, MD. John Hopkins Press, 1963, pp. 144-5.

46. Mitchener, JL, Berkowitz, B, Aguilar-Gaaxiola, S, Edgeman-Levitan, S, Lyn, M et al. *Designing new models of care for diverse communities: Why new modes of care delivery are needed*. In Cronenwett, L, Dzau, V, Culliton, B, Russell, S (eds). *Who Will Provide Primary Care and How Will They Be Trained?* Proceedings of a Conference sponsored by the Josiah Macy, Jr. Foundation, 2010. Durham, NC. Josiah Macy, Jr. Foundation, 2010, pp 84-5.

47. Geyman, JP. *Hijacked: The Road to Single Payer in the Aftermath of Stolen Health Care Reform*. Friday Harbor, WA. Copernicus Healthcare. Second edition, 2012.

48. Park, E. Allowing insurers to withhold data on enrollees' health status could undermine key part of health reform. Center on Budget and Policy Priorities. December 12, 2011.

49. Nolte, E, McKee, M. Variations in amenable mortality—Trends in 16 high-income countries. New York. The Commonwealth Fund, September 23, 2011

50. Mathews, AW. The future of U.S. health care. *Wall Street Journal*, December 12, 2011: B 1.

The Promise:
PAY YOUR OWN WAY, OR THE "SAFETY NET" WILL CATCH YOU

CHAPTER 8

Securing Our Health Care Needs: Can The Markets Do It?

"In America, the over-reliance on market logic and market institutions is ruining the health-care system. Market enthusiasts fail to tabulate all the costs of relying on market forces to allocate health care—the fragmentation, opportunism, asset rearranging, overhead, under-investment in public health, and the assault on norms of service and altruism. They assume either a degree of self-regulation that the health markets cannot generate, or far-sighted public supervision that contradicts the rest of their world view. Health care now consumes fully one-seventh of our entire national income. There is nor realm of our mixed economy where markets yield more perverse results."[1]

—Robert Kuttner, co-founder of the Economic Policy Institute and author of *Everything for Sale: The Virtues and Limits of Markets*, 1999.

"In this country we are at a crossroads between Alistair Campbell's vision of health care as a shared value—something we all own and to which we all must have access—and the nightmare of a health care Third World in which a fat, bloated health care system lavishes its services on the insured rich while uninsured children and the excluded poor die of measles and polio. It seems to me that the choice is easy enough, especially in terms of what we want our legacy to be."[2]

—Emily Friedman, independent writer, teacher and
analyst on health policy and ethics.

We now have to ask whether health care markets, which claim to be able to fix all of our health care delivery problems, can also bring Americans a sense of security over their present and future health care needs. Judging from this chapter's heading, you might expect this to be a short chapter! And you are right, for this is one area not highly valued or pursued by the free market. But if you can find good examples of health care markets providing long-term security for patients, let me know!

Since a growing part of our population feels increasing worried and insecure about its ability to afford and gain access to essential care down the road, this is a matter we must address here. Most Americans are concerned about these kinds of questions for themselves and their families: can I depend on my present insurance coverage?; for those on employer-sponsored insurance (ESI), what if I lose my job?; can I keep my own doctor if my coverage changes?; will I be able to afford necessary care as prices go up and my income doesn't keep pace?; what will happen if I become disabled?; and will Medicare be here for me when I get to that age?

This chapter undertakes two main goals: (1) to summarize market ideology as it relates to these questions, and consider the extent of insecurity that results from the volatility and unreliability of markets; and (2) to ask what health security is and whether it is an achievable goal in this country?

MARKETS GIVE US VOLATILITY, UNRELIABILITY AND INSECURITY

The only reliable thing about markets in health care is that they will be *unreliable* over the years. They are more oriented to short-term profits than to service over the long-term. When sufficient profits are not achieved, they consider changing their approach or exiting the market, in either case frequently disrupting their relationships with patients and families.

To be fair, security was never the intent of markets. Free market ideology in fact calls for the opposite, as these kinds of statements clearly demonstrate:

- The new House Majority in the House brought forward a plan in 1995 to privatize Medicare, shifting it from a defined benefits to a defined contribution program; as Speaker of the House, Newt Gingrich predicted that this kind of "reform" could "solve the Medicare problem" by causing it "to wither on the vine."[3]

- As Secretary of the Treasury during George W. Bush's first term and former top executive at two large multinational corporations, Paul O'Neill proposed that corporations should be tax exempt, like churches, and that Medicare and Medicaid should be eliminated since "able-bodied adults should save enough on a regular basis so they can provide for their own retirement and, for that matter, health and medical needs."[4]

In earlier chapters we have described how deregulated health care markets pursue their financial bottom lines before service, and that long-term stability and security of their relationships with their customers is hardly a leading concern.

These examples suggest the extent of disruption engendered by everyday business practices of three major stakeholders on the supply side.

Private insurers unilaterally change their coverage policies, rates, arrangements for preferred physicians and other providers, hospitals and other facilities (increasingly, with narrowed networks restricting choice) whenever they feel those changes will earn higher profits and returns to shareholders. On many occasions, patients are forced to change physicians, disrupting previous continuity of care, and often posing difficulties in finding new physicians, especially if uninsured, underinsured, on Medicare or Medicaid. For those still covered by ESI (no more than six of ten working Americans), there are new pressing concerns, including the likelihood that their employers will decrease their own contribution, shift employees to exchanges in 2014, offer policies with increasing deductibles and policies of lower actuarial value, or terminate coverage altogether.

Even with ESI, there is a long list of reasons to feel insecure about ongoing coverage, including inability to get coverage due to one's age, family history, health status, income (to afford increasing cost-sharing), whether or not the insurer denies future claims, and new caps on benefits. The real goal of the industry is shown by its pushing for higher premiums even as it makes record profits while utilization of care drops off among its enrollees.[5]

Private insurers "earn" their profits by medical underwriting, skillfully avoiding covering the small proportion of the population that accounts for most health care costs. We know that only 5 percent of patients account for 50 percent of annual health care costs, while 10 percent account for 72 percent of health care spending.[6] With these numbers in mind, Dr. Julian Tudor Hart, experienced general practitioner and health services analyst in the United Kingdom, coined the "inverse care law" some 40 years ago, whereby the sickest people in greatest need are always the least profitable and worst served when markets control the system.[7] This is exactly the dynamic used by private insurers if they can—shift the sicker, more expensive patients to public programs if possible, thereby adding to the adverse selection already burdening these programs.

Most regulation of private health plans is done at the state level. There are three distinct parts to the regulatory apparatus—large group, small group, and individual. Since each part varies by state, the market is divided into 150 different state-level markets. The industry maintains a strong lobbying presence in state houses across the country, enabling them to maneuver around state regulators with some agility, as these examples show:

- They shop among states for those with the least onerous regulations in each of these markets.[8]
- When large employers are mandated to offer new benefits, they may fall back on their exemption under the Employment Retirement Income and Security Act (ERISA) or drop coverage altogether.[9]
- Insurers can circumvent state regulations by forming a group to which the insurer issues a master group policy, then selling individual certificates under the master policy across state lines.[10]
- When states try to increase access to mental health services, health plans that were providing such coverage may impose new restrictions, such as cutting coverage by visit time or days per year, or stopping all mental health coverage.[11]

In mid-December 2011, the insurance industry got a surprise Christmas present from the federal government. HHS issued a ruling that gave the states the authority to determine how "essential health benefits" will be defined. States will have discretion to determine the scope of benefits to be required of insurers in their states. The ACA lists 10 categories of essential benefits that should be offered in the small-group and individual markets:

- ambulatory patient services
- emergency services
- hospitalization
- maternity and newborn care
- mental health and substance use disorder services, including behavioral health treatment
- prescription drugs
- rehabilitative and habilitative services and devices
- laboratory services
- preventive and wellness services and chronic disease management
- pediatric services, including oral and vision care[12]

But the HHS ruling avoids mandating details of what services must be provided in each category, leaving a high degree of discretion to the states. States are free to choose among typical plans offered by any of these insurers—the three largest state employee health plans, one of the three largest federal employee health plan options, or the largest HMO plan offered in the state's commercial market.[13] We can expect all this to result in the leanest of minimal benefit packages in most states, more in the interest of insurers than patients.

When private insurers take over public programs, they exploit them and fail to cut costs as they claim. Instead they cut services and exit the market if they can't make sufficient profits. Between 1999 and 2002, for example, about one-third of Medicare + Choice enrollees were abandoned across the country when their plans left their counties. For-profit plans of large national corporations were two and one-half times more likely to leave the market than not-for-profit insurers.[14] Humana, as the biggest private Medicare Advantage program with revenue gains increasing from $271 million in 2008 to $474 million in 2009, was already eyeing more lucrative markets in specialty biotech drugs and chronic disease management programs.[15] WellPoint gives us a more recent example of its lack of commitment to enrollees. After a drop in its fourth-quarter 2011 profits in its Medicare Advantage program in Northern California, due to unexpectedly high costs for seniors' care,

WellPoint walked away from that "problem" market. Its CEO, Angela Braly, said simply: "We believe we have taken the appropriate actions to improve our senior business results for 2012."[16]

In Florida, privatized Medicaid plans in the mid-1990s were a disaster—up to 50 percent of their funding was diverted to overhead and profits, with widespread fraud and abuse exposed by a series of articles by investigative reporters Fred Schulte and Jenni Bergal in the *Florida Sun Sentinel*.[17] Today, privatized Medicaid programs are still being sold to various states as cost containment initiatives despite their poor track record. After that expose of Medicaid fraud, per capita Medicaid spending in Florida rose much more slowly between 2001 and 2009 than private coverage by large employers (up 30 percent vs. 112 percent, respectively).[18]

Employers. Under increasing pressure of the costs of health care making it difficult for them to compete and stay afloat, employers shift more of their costs for ESI to their employees, move away from defined benefits to defined contributions, increase deductibles and cost-sharing, and eliminate retiree coverage. Some consider dropping coverage altogether.

A 2010 report by *Fortune* magazine, based upon internal documents of large companies such as AT&T and Verizon, found that many are considering dumping their ESI in exchange for paying the penalties imposed by the government under ACA.[19] And a growing number of employers are looking for ways to shift the responsibility for their workers' coverage to health insurance exchanges when they become operational in 2014. Other employers offer insurance that is nearly meaningless, such at the policy offered by McDonald's Corp. with annual limits of only $2,000 (which was even approved by the federal Department of Health and Human Services).[20] Such "coverage" does not compute when we consider that the average costs today for cardiac bypass surgery or a hip replacement run in the neighborhood of $45,000.

Hospitals. Activities among hospitals, especially as they gear up for accountable care organizations (ACOs) under the ACA, add further to the insecurity of patients, families and communities. As they chase potential new revenue streams in a changing environment, many hospitals are building systems targeting well-insured patients. Mergers among hospitals are on the increase, and many are building networks of free-standing emergency rooms and urgent care clinics as feeders to their main hospital. As the competitive marketplace heats up, many hospitals are actively recruiting patients to come to their ERs, even for non-emergency reasons. HCA, the largest for-profit hospital chain in the country, has launched a major ER marketing campaign in Virginia, Florida, Texas and other states, using billboards advertising short wait times and other amenities. Dallas-based Tenet Healthcare Corp, another large investor-owned hospital chain, is promoting its ERs for "primary care." These visits become a cash cow for hospitals, with charges three or four times those billed in physicians' offices. They also build referrals for inpatient care and stress payers' budgets. Concerned about increasing costs of so-called emergency care, Medicaid officials in Washington State have issued new rules tightening up on hospitals' qualifying for Medicaid bonus payments for ER visits for such primary care problems as diabetes.[21]

In some cases, we are even seeing new joint arrangements between insurers and hospitals. One example is Aetna's jointly marketed plan with Banner Health, a not-for-profit 23-hospital system based in Phoenix, Arizona. Such arrangements offer both parties the possibility of larger market shares in their respective areas., and are likely to disrupt previous preferred choices of patients and perhaps physicians.[22]

Some not-for-profit hospitals with long traditions of service to their communities are packing up and moving to more affluent areas. Alan Sager, professor of health policy and management at Boston University, has studied hospital closures in 52 large and mid-sized U.S. cities over almost five decades. He has found that the most likely hospitals to shut their doors are for-profit hospitals, non-teaching hospitals, and those located in neighborhoods with high minority populations, unfortunately areas of very high medical needs.[23]

WHAT IS HEALTH CARE SECURITY
AND IS IT AN ACHIEVABLE GOAL?

American families know how to define feeling secure about their own health care. And they know all too well how it feels to be vulnerable to the next accident or major illness. In its purest form, health care security means never seeing a bill, never worrying about having to pay before receiving care, always gaining access to care regardless of age, pre-existing condition, or having a job. It means confronting disease when it happens, being free to focus on the medical issues, not the financial ones. This level of security may sound utopian and seem to be totally non-achievable, but many other advanced countries around the world either have it or something close to it.

Despite a long-standing consensus in other advanced countries around the world that health care is a human right, there is no such consensus in this country. After decades of not dealing with this question, Social Darwinism holds sway, based on ability to pay instead of medical need.

As we saw in Chapter 1, our society in this Second Gilded Age is more divided over income and class than ever, to the point that that the Occupy movement is attempting to empower the interests of the 99 percent against the ruling 1 percent. Even as health care costs soar out of sight and as our own health security becomes increasingly threatened, many Americans still can't accept that we are all in the same boat. But it doesn't take but one heart attack or car accident for a member of the one percent to realize that he or she *is* in the same boat with all of us— if the nearest ER is on divert status because of overcrowding with other urgent and emergency problems, the stakes rise quickly.

As is clear from earlier chapters, the health care "system," based as it is on markets, is the only boat we have, and it is sinking. We are told by politicians and health policy "experts" (often supported by corporate stakeholders) that the ACA which they crafted will solve our problems. We are evolving quickly into a multi-tiered health care system, with an enormous population of Americans dispossessed of even basic medical care. We need soon to decide this question of universal access and whether we really want social justice in health care.

It's not as if this question has not been seriously addressed over the years. It has, but so far to little avail in practice in this country.

In 1948, health care was recognized as a right as part of the Universal Declaration of Human Rights as adopted by the General Assembly of the United Nations. Article 25 of that document held that:

"Everyone has the right to a standard of living adequate for the health and well-being of himself and his family, including food, clothing, housing and *medical care* and necessary social services, and the right to security in the event of unemployment, *sickness*, disability, widowhood, old age or other lack of livelihood in circumstances beyond his control."[24]

The right to health care was later adopted by the World Health Organization (WHO) in its *Declaration on the Rights of Patients*.[25]

In 1999, an international working group from the U.S. and three other countries (the UK, Mexico and South Africa) endorsed the concept of health care as a human right. Known as the Tavistock Group, it included physicians, nurses, academicians, ethicists, health care executives, a jurist, an economist, and a philosopher.[26]

In 2004, the IOM's Committee on the Consequences of Uninsurance proposed this set of principles:

1. "Coverage should be universal.
2. Coverage should be continuous.
3. Coverage should be affordable for individuals and families.
4. Strategy should be affordable and sustainable for society.
5. Coverage should enhance health through high-quality care."[27]

But these high goals fall prey to the political process of distortion, denial and disinformation across a wide political spectrum. Many, if not most market advocates reject in principle the idea of health care as a human right. Clearly, the right to health care must be qualified if it is to have meaning and sustainability for any health care system. Larry Churchill, well-known ethicist at the Vanderbilt University, gives us this useful perspective:

"There is a moral right to health care, but not of the sort often claimed. It is a right grounded not in purchasing power, merit, or social worth, but in human need. The right to health care finds its rationale in a social concept of the self, in a sense of common humanity, and in a knowledge of common vulnerability to disease and death... A right to health care is not a license to demand care. It is not a right to the very best available, or even to all one may need. Some very pressing health needs may have to be neglected because meeting them would be unreasonable in the light of other health needs or social priorities." And further: "A just health care system, whatever its final shape, requires a recognition of our sociality and mutual vulnerability to disease and death."[28]

Unfortunately, the ongoing political debate over the future of U.S. health care has become lost in demagoguery focused on peripheral issues. Fundamental issues, such as who is the health care system for and are we committed to universal access, are being carefully avoided. Our "centrist" politics of the day are being held hostage by market interests buying their perpetuation of the free market in health care. T. R. Reid, experienced reporter for the *Washington Post* both here and overseas and author of the excellent book *The Healing of America: A Global Quest for Better, Cheaper, and Fairer Health Care*, puts it this way:

"When it comes to the essential task of providing health care for people, the mighty USA is a fourth-rate power . . . [Our country never made a fundamental moral decision] to provide medical care for everybody who needs it."[29]

Theodore Marmor, professor emeritus of public policy at Yale University and Jerry Mashaw, professor of law at Yale, give us this historical perspective of how the language of our political leaders has changed from the 1930s to the present time—from

"a morally resonant language of people, family and shared social concern to the cold technical idiom of budgetary accounting... [And further]:
In 1934, the government was us. We had shared circumstances, shared risks and shared obligations. Today the government is the other—not an institution for the achievement of our common goals, but an alien presence that stands between us and the realization of individual ambitions. Programs of social insurance have become 'entitlements', a word apparently meant to signify not a collectively provided and cherished basis for family-income security but a sinister threat to our national well-being."[30]

Against this background, can we ever hope to achieve universal access to health care in this country? The lofty pronouncements of prestigious groups ring hollow as politics of the day hold us hostage on this crucial question. Well-funded "leadership" throughout the medical-industrial complex fights to avoid a larger role of government as would be obviously required to rein in markets in the public interest. We will return to this question in the last chapter, but for now, let's turn to the next chapter to consider how ethical the unfettered markets are in health care.

References

1. Kuttner, R. *Everything for Sale: The Virtues and Limits of Markets*, Chicago. University of Chicago Press, 1999, p. 140.
2. Friedman, E. Prevention, public health, and managed care: Obstacles and opportunities. *Am J Prev Med* 14 (3 suppl): 102-5, 1998.
3. Smith, DG. *Entitlement Politics: Medicare and Medicaid 1995-2001.* New York. Aldine de Gruyter, 2002: 71, citing *Congressional Quarterly Almanac*, 1995, pp. 7-13.
4. Hartmann, T. *Unequal Protection: The Rise of Corporate Dominance and the Theft of Human Rights.* Emmaus, PA. Rodale Press, 2002, pp.177-8.
5. Abelson, R. Health insurers making record profits as many postpone care. *New York Times*, May 13, 2011.
6. Physicians for a National Health Program (PNHP). Chicago, IL. Available at www.pnhp.org, 2002.
7. Hart, JT. The Inverse Care Law. 1: 405-12, 1971.
8. Hall, M. The geography of health insurance regulation: A guide to identifying, exploiting, and policing market boundaries. *Health Affairs (Millwood)* 19 (2) 173-82, 2000.
9. Kleinke, JD. *Oxymorons: The myths of the U.S. health care system.* San Francisco. Jossey-Bass, 2001, p. 189.
10. Ibid # 8.
11. Frank, RG, Kovanagi, C, McGuire, TG. The politics and economics of mental health "parity" laws. *Health Affairs (Millwood)* 16 (4):108, 1997.
12. Pear, R. Health care law will let states tailor benefits. *New York Times*, December 17, 2001: A1.
13. Clark, CS. HHS proposes rule to help define essential health benefits.

Government Executive, December 16, 2011.

14. Lake, T, Brown, R. *Medicare + Choice Withdrawals: Understanding Key Factors*. Menlo Park, CA. Kaiser Family Foundation, June 2002.

15. Johnson, A. Humana CEO keeps eye on health care reform signposts ahead. *Wall Street Journal*, November 23, 2009: B1.

16. Kamp, J. Care for seniors saps WellPoint profit. *Wall Street Journal*, January 20, 2012: B8.

17. Schulte, F, Bergal, J. *Profits from Pain: Florida's Medicaid HMOs*. Five-part series in the *Florida Sun Sentinel*, 1994.

18. Mellowe, G. Florida Center for Fiscal and Economic Policy, April 1, 2011.

19. Adamy, J, Johnson, A. Rules eased for some health plans. *Wall Street Journal*, November 23, 2010: B1.

20. Tully, S. Documents reveal AT&T, Verizon, others thought about dropping employer-sponsored benefits. *Fortune.* May 6, 2010.

21. Galewitz, P. As hospitals push ERs, states' Medicaid budgets pressured. *Kaiser Health News*, August 22, 2011.

22. Mathews, AW. The future of U.S. health care. *Wall Street Journal*, December 12, 2011: B1.

23. Sager, A. With hospitals, it's survival of the fattest, not the fittest. Report from the Robert Wood Johnson Foundation, January 2001. Available at htpp://www.rwjf.org/reports/grr/028054.htm

24. Adopted by the General Assembly on 10 December 1948. Printed in: von Munch, I, Buske, A (eds). *International Law the Essential Treaties and Other Relevant Documents*. 1985: 435ff.

25. Carmi, A. On patients' rights. *Med Law* 10 (1): 77-82, 1991.

26. The Tavistock Group. A shared statement of ethical principles for those who shape and give health care: a working draft. *Effective Clin Pract* 2 (3): 143-5, 1999/

27. Committee on the Consequences of Uninsurance. Institute of Medicine. *Insuring America's Health: Principles and Recommendations.* National Academies Press. Washington, D.C. 150-1, 2004.

28. Churchill, LR. *Rationing Health Care in America: Perceptions and Principles of Justice.* Notre Dame, IN. University of Notre Dame 90, 91,94-6,135, 1987.)

29. Reid, TR. *The Healing of America: A Global Quest for Better, Cheaper, and Fairer Health Care.* New York. Penguin Press, 2009.

30. Marmor, TR, Mashaw, JL. How do you say 'economic security'? *New York Times*, September 23, 2011.

The Promise:
FREE MARKETS ARE SELF-REGULATING

CHAPTER 9

Markets, Slippery Ethics, and the Invisible Hand in Health Care

The power of the "invisible hand" as a self-regulating force in markets first appeared in the writings of Adam Smith in the 18th century. Since then the term has been elaborated upon by many economists and adopted as a quasi-religious belief by advocates of the free market for its claimed beneficial effects on society. Despite its failures in housing, financial and other markets in recent years, conservative economists still worship at the altar of the invisible hand as a guiding force out of the wilderness.

This chapter has two goals: (1) to briefly describe the history of this concept, its supposed benefits and limitations; and (2) to look for the invisible hand's workings in our health care system.

MARKET WORSHIP OF THE INVISIBLE HAND

For all the attribution and credit given to Adam Smith for the invisible hand metaphor by advocates of *laissez faire* economics, he mentioned the idea only three times in his writings. The idea has been seized upon and further developed by those promoting free markets as an effective way to channel self-interest toward socially desirable ends. [1]

In his excellent recent book, *The Golden Calf: Economism and American Policy*, Dr. Howard Brody, family physician, bioethicist and philosopher based at the University of Texas in Galveston, explores the history of *economism*, a belief system holding that the "free market" should be allowed to control as much of our lives and society as possible without the interference of government. He traces its historical roots from evangelism in nineteenth century England and the "Protestant Ethic" that evolved from eighteenth century Calvinist and Puritan beliefs in America. Brody also reveals that Adam Smith was a social and political philosopher who recognized the limits of free markets to regulate themselves, and that a whole society has to be working well for markets to function well.[2] Brody points to the work of Sankar Muthu, associate professor of political science at the University of Chicago and author of *Enlightenment Against Empire*, who notes that Smith was harshly critical about the harmful effects of international joint stock trading companies in the 18th century, believing them to be unjust and cruel to those over whom they had power. As Muthu observed 1n 2008:

> "Given Smith's belief in the fundamental sociability of human beings, the sociability of commerce both within and across societies simply puts into practice a core feature of what it means to be human. Thus, when commerce becomes thwarted, subjected to the power of a few, and restricted to a wealthy elite, the consequences are not only materially damaging for domestic economies and international markets, but they are also, in a fundamental sense, dehumanizing."[3]

As philosopher Alan Wolfe has written, markets as late as the early 1800s were almost entirely local, within which they met face-to-face, forged stronger interpersonal ties, gained respect for their neighbors, and helped to build a sense of community. In that context, the invisible hand may have played a significant role. Market transactions were more personal, helped to support sustainable norms of beneficial social conduct, and unscrupulous sellers would pay a high price for deceiving buyers.[4]

But today's marketplace in this global economy run by distant multi-national corporations and the 1 percent of our society is a whole different world—impersonal, non-transparent, and often without recourse to unfair business practices.Meanwhile, free market ideology lives on under government policies largely dictated by the power and money of the corporate elite.

Margaret R. Somers, professor of history and sociology at the University of Michigan and author of *Genealogies of Citizenship: Markets, Statelessness, and the Right to Have Rights*, writes about the corrupting effects of economism on our democracy:

> "Three decades of what has become market-driven governance are transforming growing numbers of once rights-bearing citizens into socially excluded internally rightless and stateless persons. A political culture that tolerates, even legitimates, these brute disparities in life chances has a corrosive effect not only on citizenship and human rights, but equally on perceptions of what we owe each other as fellow humans."[5]

Joseph E. Stiglitz, former chief economist at the World Bank, cuts to the heart of the matter with this incisive insight:

> "Unlike his followers, Adam Smith was aware of some of the limitations of free markets, and research since then has further clarified why free markets, by themselves, often do not lead to what is best. As I put it in my new book, *Making Globalization Work*, the reason that the invisible hand often seems invisible is that it is often not there... Government plays an important role in banking and securities regulation, and a host of other areas: some regulation is required to make markets work."[6]

Despite the obvious limitations of the free market in health care, many economists, conservative ideologues, and policymakers keep telling us that the invisible hand will work. Here is one example, among many, by Dr. Robert M. Sade, professor of surgery at the Medical University of South Carolina, who maintains that::

> "The history of this country's health care system and the experiences of other nations provide evidence of the superiority of free markets in reaching for the goals of universal access, control of costs, and sustaining the quality of health care."[7]

But if we look at how health care has been transformed by deregulated markets over the last thirty to forty years in this country, we now find fragmentation, depersonalization with patients now viewed as consumers and physicians and other health professionals as providers, lack of transparency and accountability, and corporate interests on the supply side serving their own self-interest over the public interest. Increasingly employed by business interests in health care, the medical profession has rightly lost autonomy, stature and trust. And government has fallen far short of assuring Americans access to quality health care that is affordable. This is how Dr. Carl Elliott, physician, philosopher and professor at the Center for Bioethics at the University of Minnesota, sums up our current quandary:

"Without actually intending it, we have constructed a medical system in which deception is often not just tolerated but rewarded. A series of social and legislative changes have transformed medicine into a business, yet because of medicine's history as a self-regulating profession, no one is really policing it. On the surface, our medical system looks very similar to the way it looked twenty-five years ago, Dig deeper, though, and you can see the same patterns of misconduct emerging again and again."[8]

With this background, let's go looking for the invisible hand helping us in health care!

WHERE IS THE INVISIBLE HAND IN HEALTH CARE MARKETS?

Here we will take a broad look at the major players on the supply side of U.S. health care, looking for patterns based on readily available reports. While I've tried hard to find examples of the invisible hand actually working in the patient's best interests (e.g. for more available, less expensive care of high quality based on competition) acting in the manner that was visualized in local markets two centuries ago, the hand is nowhere in sight. Instead, we don't have to look far to understand what is going on, and who is best being served.

As we saw in Chapter 3, the medical-industrial-complex is filled with sharp business practices that push boundaries between acceptable business practices (a very low bar!) and unethical practices. But in none of those instances could we find an invisible hand serving the interests of patients and their families. Let's take another brief tour across major players in the market-based health care "system", starting this time with physicians, since they order most of what is done in health care and have "professed" themselves to put the interests of their patients first.

Physicians.

The practice of medicine has undergone an enormous transformation over the last thirty to forty years—from a cottage industry based on traditional values of service to a less autonomous, increasingly employed status within corporate systems. The service ethic has been seriously eroded as the business "ethic" overruns it. Many physicians have resisted this transformation, many others have become comfortable with it, and some have exploited it. As a result, the profession's traditional commitment to service, ethical standards, professionalism, and to the patient's interest above all else have been called into question.[9] The extent of this erosion is reflected in the public attitudes toward physicians. A 1999 study of major social institutions in the U.S. found that public confidence in physicians dropped from 50 percent in 1987 to about 22 percent in 1999.[10]

Some medical organizations have attempted to reverse the damaging impacts of financial conflicts of interest (COIs) on professionalism, including the AMA through its Council on Ethical and Judicial Affairs, the Accreditation Council for Continuing Medical Education, and the American College of Physicians. But their guidelines, well intended as they are, generally have no mechanisms to codify transgressions and lack teeth. The failure of most medical organizations to regulate themselves and discipline their members has led Dr. David Rothman, professor of social medicine and Director of the Center for the Study of Society and Medicine at Columbia College of Physicians and Surgeons, to this conclusion:

> "The inadequacies of self-regulation make it clear that an exam-
> ination of professionalism must go beyond questions of money
> and managed care. To the extent that self-regulation is the focus,
> professionalism today has to be invented, not restored."[11]

Dr. David Lotto, a psychoanalytic historian, gives us this further insight:

"There are far too many health professionals among us who are willing to bend, contort, and turn inside out, our traditional professional values. Too many are willing to accommodate to the values of the corporate world where protecting the wealth of those who are paying you becomes a legitimate part of your professional function. Making this kind of accommodation has its rewards: mainly financial security and a comfortable middle class lifestyle. But like all such Faustian bargains, there is a steep price to pay. The problem is that in order to avoid anxiety and guilt we come to share the moral blind spots of our corporate culture."[12]

These further examples reveal that any attempts by the profession to regulate itself fall far short of the mark, and that much of the house of medicine is still being controlled by larger business interests beholden to the standard investor agenda of making money at any cost.

- *Financial ties to industry*. A 2007 survey of U.S. physicians found that 94 percent report some kind of relationship with the drug industry, ranging from gifts from sales representatives to dinners and trips to resort locations for conferences; 35 percent were paid as speakers or consultants.[13]
- *Deceptive and misleading advice*. Presidents of two major U.S. plastic surgery organizations—the American Society of Plastic Surgeons and the American Society for Aesthetic Plastic Surgery—advised their members in a 2011 members-only webinar to avoid using the word "cancer" when talking to patients and the media about a rare kind of cancer occurring in some women who had received breast implants. Although the FDA had earlier called attention to a possible link between breast implants and anaplastic large cell lymphoma (ALCL), a rare malignant cancer, the president of one of these organizations asked members to refer to ALCL as a "condition" in order not to alarm patients. The FDA has found a total of 34 cases of ALCL in breast implant patients worldwide, one-half of them requiring chemotherapy,

radiation therapy or a combination of both. A concerned plastic surgeon reported this incident to Public Citizen, which followed up with the FDA and led the organizations to take this webinar offline.[14]

- **Under-reporting of risks**. Medtronic, the giant medical device maker, has sponsored 13 clinical trials in recent years of its product, Infuse Bone Graft, used in spinal surgery. A 2011 full-issue report by *The Spine Journal* revealed that peer-reviewed industry-supported journal publications greatly underestimated the risks of serious complications, including cancer, male sterility, infections, bone dissolution, and worsened back and leg pain. These risks are 10 to 50 times higher than originally reported.[15] The median amount of Medtronic money going to researchers over these years ranged from $12 million to $16 million, most of which went to just a few participating surgeons. Although the FDA approved Infuse for one type of spine surgery in 2002, at least 85 percent of its use is now off-label for unapproved uses, representing about $900 million in annual revenue for Medtronic. Both the Senate Finance Committee and the Department of Justice have been investigating this matter.[16]

- **Institutional review boards (IRBs)** are committees charged with overseeing ethical standards for medical research in this country. As described by Elliott in his previous mentioned book *White Coat Black Hat*, many are commercial, for-profit operations that are a lucrative and non-transparent business. As an example, a GAO sting operation several years ago exposed Coast IRB, based in Colorado Springs, CO that had rejected only one of 356 research protocols over a five-year period. It had advertised itself as a rapid turn-around committee that offered "speed, quality and service, guided by the light of ethics," further advising drug companies that even a single day's delay of a fifty-center Phase III drug trial could cost the sponsor $6 million. It had offered drug companies coupons inviting them to "coast through your next study." In its sting operation, the GAO had drawn up a totally unacceptable proposal, including a forged and long-outdated medical license of the "researcher" as lead investigator, but the proposal still received prompt approval by the IRB. Commercial

IRBs have an obvious conflict of interest—the more protocols they approve, the more money they make, and the more their business grows.[17,18]

- *Financial COIs* between physicians and industry sponsors often go undisclosed, even when physicians as consultants and authors make more than $1 million a year from industry. Journals that publish their subsequent articles also frequently fail to disclose these COIs, according to a 2010 study by a team of researchers at Columbia University with support by the Institute of Medicine as a Profession (IMAP).[19] Commenting on the study, Dr. Marcia Angell, former editor of the *New England Journal of Medicine* and author of *The Truth about the Drug Companies: How They Deceive Us and What to Do About It*, had this to say:

> "It is one more indication of the widespread corruption of the medical profession by industry money."[20]

Beyond the sharp and often shady business practices of other major players in our market-based system, these are more examples where the invisible hand is nowhere to be seen.

Insurers.

- *Discount health plans.* This is a new product that targets a growing group of uninsured and underinsured Americans. Patients pay a monthly or annual fee to get a card that gives access to a network that is supposed to offer reduced charges for physician visits, prescription drugs and other services, such as eye glasses. Patients pay all of these costs up front, less whatever discount has been negotiated with the plan. But many of the networks have few providers, discounts can be much less than advertised, and some of these plans are not legitimate. State regulators are beginning to crack down on their unethical practices.[21]
- *Anti-competitive agreements*. An antitrust lawsuit has recently been filed in a number of states alleging that Blue Cross Blue Shield companies and hospitals have raised hospital prices. In Michigan, for example, Blue Cross negotiated contracts with 70 of the state's 131 general acute-care hospitals that then charged

rival insurers 30 to 40 percent higher charges than Blue Cross. The U.S. Department of Justice is investigating the matter.[22]

Hospitals.

- *Sales reps' bonuses.* A growing number of hospitals around the country are now hiring former drug and medical device sales representatives to visit physicians' offices in an effort to attract admissions of their patients to their hospitals over competing facilities. Hospitals are mining data to find which physicians have the most profitable, best-insured patients, then send their sales reps that way. HCA Inc and Tenet Healthcare Corp, the nation's largest and third largest investor-owned hospital chains, respectively, with well-known records of unethical practices, each have some 150 "physician liaisons" working as sales reps, who can make tens of thousands of dollars in bonuses if physicians increase referrals to their hospitals.[23]
- *Industry-supported adoption of medical devices.* This is another murky area involving large payments to selected physicians as consultants to industry in an effort to have their hospitals adopt their products. As just one example, the University Medical Center of Southern Nevada in Las Vegas, adopted Biotronic defibrillators after the hospital's cardiologists received large consulting payments from the company. Later, the hospital claimed improved outcomes for its cardiac patients, without releasing supportive data, when in fact these outcomes cannot be accurately known due to the shortcomings of the National Cardiovascular Data Registry, an ICD registry.[24]
- *Marketing of back surgery in small hospitals.* Some small hospitals in California "specialize" in spinal fusion surgery for workman's compensation patients, a group that many other hospitals don't want to accept due to questions about payment and legal issues. Pacific Medical Center of Long Beach and its close neighbor, Tri-City Regional Hospital just 8 miles away, are under investigation by federal authorities in Los Angeles for performing record numbers of spinal fusion procedures and recruiting surgeons to perform them with kickbacks of $15,000 to $20,000 per procedure. These have allegedly been paid by over-billing the costs of the spinal fusion hardware by two to ten

times their actual purchase price. The distributor and business management consultant arranging all this for Tri-City, a non-profit institution, was paid more than $3 million between 2008 and 2011, during which Tri-Cities billings for spinal surgery soared twenty-fold to $65 million. The case is still unsettled at this writing.[25]

Home Health Care.
- *Gaming Medicare coverage.* Medicare reimbursement for home health care services depend in part on the number of therapy visits each patient receives. With the intent to assure patients necessary home care, Medicare changed its reimbursement policy in 2008. Instead of offering home care companies bonuses of a few thousand dollars upon reaching a 10-visit threshold, other thresholds for smaller bonuses were set at 6, 14 and 20 visits. After this change, bonuses paid to the home health care industry went up 19 percent at the 6-visit level, by 42 percent at 14 visits, and by 30 percent at 20 visits, while declining by 43 percent at the prior 10-visit level, according to CMS data.[26]

Drug industry.
- *Direct to consumer advertising (DTC)*, though banned in many other countries, has burgeoned in the U.S. since the late 1990s, typically hyping the benefits of drugs while downplaying their risks. Together with drug Web sites and online drug sales, DTC has led to exponential increases in drug sales and profits, often by selling us new "diseases" (e.g. seasonal allergies, erectile dysfunction, and low testosterone) and even the *risk* of disease (e.g. osteopenia for osteoporosis). Dr. Larry Schneiderman, physician and bioethicist at the University of California San Diego, notes how well the movement toward patient autonomy coincides with corporate interests to sell their products.[27] DTC encourages patients to engage in self-diagnosis, and to seek specific medicines from their physicians, who often respond to their requests.[28]
- *Accelerated FDA reviews.* Our "user fee" system of regulation was enacted in 1992 with the passage of the Prescription Drug User Fee Act (PDUFA). Industry now pays for more than one-

half of the FDA's budget, representing an ongoing "fox in the hen house" conflict of interest. Industry provides funding for additional reviewers, has clout in renegotiating new terms every five years, and keeps pushing for accelerated reviews. These drug reviews are often based on short-term or surrogate markers without requiring evidence of real clinical improvement. As a result of this industry-friendly regulatory system, it is estimated that at least 20 million Americans were exposed to drugs approved in the early years of PDUFA that were later withdrawn after their serious adverse effects were recognized.[29]

- **Drug advertising in medical journals** is a major funding source for most clinical journals. Drug companies have been known to withdraw advertising from those journals that seem opposed to their interests. Published articles that underreport their drugs' toxic side effects can bring journals large profits (e.g. Merck paid the *New England Journal of Medicine* $900,000 for one article).[30]

- **PhRMA's ethical code as window dressing.** In response to growing criticism of its business practices, PhRMA, the industry's trade group, has attempted to quiet ethical concerns with its Code on Interactions with Healthcare Professionals, which asserts that its main goal is exchange of educational and scientific information between industry and the medical profession. While making some minor proposals for change, the Code remains entirely voluntary, and lacks mechanisms for assuring compliance. In his 2010 book *The Risks of Prescription Drugs*, Donald Light sums up the current situation this way: "The new Code looks more like window dressing in front of the ongoing commercialization of professional judgment."[31]

- **Illegal distribution of narcotic drugs.** In February 2012 the Drug Enforcement Administration (DEA) blocked four pharmacies in Sanford, FL, including two CVS locations, from selling controlled substances. At the same time, the DEA moved to punish Cardinal Health Inc, the second largest pharmaceutical distributor in the country, with revenue in 2011 of more than $100 billion. In 2011, Cardinal Health shipped enough oxycodone to Sanford to give 59 of these narcotic pills to every man, woman, and child there! The DEA reported that Cardinal Health supplied the four pharmacies with 50 times the volume of oxycodone shipped to the average Florida pharmacy. All of these companies denied any wrongdoing. This is not a new problem for Cardinal Health—it paid a $34 million fine in 2008 to settle allegations that it had failed to prevent supplies from being diverted.

This practice has spawned a huge and deadly black market. According to the Centers for Disease Control and Prevention (CDC), the numbers of annual deaths from overdoses of narcotic drugs has nearly quadrupled over a ten-year period, even surpassing deaths from traffic accidents in some states. On the street, black market prices for oxycodone are about $15 to $20 per pill, compared to less than $1 for a legitimate prescription.[32]

Medical Devices.
- *Specialty society-industry "partnership" for implantable defibrillators.* A 2011 report by *ProPublica* and *USA Today* described the incestuous relationships between the Heart Rhythm Society (with 5,100 members) and manufacturers of cardiac defibrillators. Large sums of money flow to the Society (almost one-half of the $16 million collected in 2010), most of its directors have financial COIs with industry, and marketing promotional blitzes are a main feature at its annual meetings. These relationships have led to the overuse of defibrillators, and have drawn the interest of the Senate Judiciary Committee.[33] A 2011 report in the *Journal of the American Medical Association* found that 22.5 percent of patientsreceiving implantable defibrillators did not need them.[34]
- *Overseas marketing of hip implants rejected by FDA.* The DePuy orthopedic division of the health care products giant Johnson & Johnson continued to market its defective all-metal ASR hip replacement overseas even after the FDA had rejected it due to high premature failure rates. The company also continued to sell a closely related implant in this country through a regulatory loophole not requiring evidence of safety and effectiveness. The company finally recalled these devices after failure rates continued to grow both here and abroad. There are now some 5,000 lawsuits pending against the company involving some patients crippled by the shedding of tiny particles of metallic

debris from these implants. While there is no evidence that laws were broken, where were the CEOs and boards of directors who permitted the ongoing sales of these defective products?[35]

Marketing posing as research.
- *Useless studies.* Phase IV drug studies give us classic example of conflicts of interests between physician prescribers and drug manufacturers wanting to market their products. They are not encumbered by rigorous overview by IRB's, many of which are also for-profit and are being paid by the drug companies that produced the drugs being studied. The FDA has already approved the drugs, and does not monitor Phase IV trials. "seeding trials" are one example of this kind of for-profit "research." They are typically run by drug companies' marketing departments, which invite several hundreds of physicians to participate, hoping that they will become high prescribers as they become more familiar with the drug being "studied." While not illegal, these "studies" operate under the radar without any federal human subject protections.[36] One notorious example is the 12-year seeding trial of Neurontin, a seizure drug made by Pfizer. As shown by a scathing 2011 report in the *Archives of Internal Medicine*, researchers were inexperienced and untrained, and the research design was so flawed as to render any conclusions meaningless. More importantly, 11 patients died during the study and 73 more had serious adverse events. These were not publicized. Later litigation documents confirmed that it was more marketing than research.[37]

MISSING IN ACTION: THE INVISIBLE HAND

This brief tour of the big players in our medical-industrial-complex fails to find Adam Smith's supposed invisible hand making markets work in the best interests of patients and their families on the receiving end of U.S. health care. The business 'ethic' is in charge and we find that the ethical pronouncements within the medical profession and among the corporate stakeholders are more self-serving and unenforceable, and fall way short of the public interest. While most of these practices are legal, they do not give us the confidence about health care that we want and deserve. But it gets worse, as we will see in the next chapter, where we also find widespread fraud.

We can see how the invisible hand can really work for many commodities, products such as a car or a computer. In those instances, buyers can develop sophisticated experience and preferences that can exert market power over the suppliers. But, as we have seen here, this just doesn't work in health care.

Patients are faced with how best to navigate our complex health care system for their own specific medical needs. They find it difficult to shop for the best value, are often pressed by the urgency of their problems, are limited by their ability to pay and resources available to them, and accurate information about their alternatives is usually not available. In short, patients cannot exert aggregate consumer choice as a market force. Moreover, most decisions about what health care professional to see and which hospital to use are made by their physicians.

Throughout this chapter we have seen how the ideal of the invisible hand doesn't work its magic in health care, especially where greed prevails on the supply side of the health care business. But greed isn't our only problem, not the only force that has supplanted the service ethic. In the next chapter we review an even more corrosive force—fraud—which further invalidates any hope that that markets can deliver the best health care.

References

1. Wikipedia, Invisible hand. December 14, 2011.
2. Brody, H. *The Golden Calf: Economism and American Policy.* Friday Harbor, WA. Copernicus Health Care, 2011.
3. Muthu, S. Adam Smith's critique of international trading companies: theorizing "globalization" in the Age of Enlightenment. *Political Theory* 36: 185-212, 2008. p. 192.
4. Wolfe, A. *Whose Keeper? Social Science and Moral Obligation.* Berkeley, CA. University of California Press, 1989: 19.
5. Somers, MR. *Genealogies of Citizenship: Markets, Statelessness, and the Right to Have Rights.* New York. Cambridge University Press, 2008, p.3.
6. Stiglitz, JE. As quoted in Altman, D. *Managing Globalization.* In Q & *Answers* with Joseph E. Stiglitz, Columbia University and *The International Herald Tribune*, October 11, 2006.

7. Sade, RM. Foundational ethics of the health care system: The moral and practical superiority of free market reforms. *Journal of Medicine and Philosophy* 33: 461-97, 2008.

8. Elliott, C. *White Coat Black Hat: Adventures on the Dark Side of Medicine.* Boston. Beacon Press, 2010: p. xi.

9. Pescasolido, BA, Tuch, SA, Martin, JA. The profession of medicine of medicine and the public: examining America's changing confidence in physician authority from the beginning of the "Health Care Crisis" to the era of health care reform. *J Health & Soc Behavior* 42 (1): 1-16, 2001.

10. Mycek, S. We're not in Kansas anymore. *Trustee* 52: 22, 1999.

11. Rothman, DJ. Medical professionalism: focusing on the real issues. *N Engl J Med* 342 (17): 1284-6, 2000.

12. Lotto, DL. The corporate takeover of the soul of healthcare. *J Psychohistory* 26 (2): 603-9, 1998.

13. Campbell, EG, Gruen, RL, Mountford, J, Miller, LG, Cleary, PD et al. A national survey of physician-industry relationships. *N Engl J Med* 356 (17): 1743-50, 2007.

14. Blair, B. Inaccurate advice on breast implant-related cancer taken offline. *Public Citizen News* 31 (2): 1, 2011.

15. Carragee, EJ, Hurwitz, EL, Weiner, BK. A critical review of recombinant human bone morphogenetic protein 2 trials in spinal surgery: emerging safety concerns and lessons learned. *The Spine Journal* 11: 471-91, 2011.

16. Meier, B, Wilson, D. Spine experts repudiate Medtronic studies. *New York Times*, June 28, 2011.

17. Ibid # 9, pp. 158-68.

18. Mundy, A. Sting operation exposes gaps in oversight of human experiments. *Wall Street Journal*, March 26, 2009.

19. Chimonas, S, Frosch, Z, Rothman, DJ. From disclosure to transparency: the use of company payment data. *Arch Intern Med* on line, September 13, 2010.

20. Angell, M as quoted by Wilson, D. Medical industry ties often undisclosed in journals. *New York Times*, September 14, 2010: B1.

21. Mertens, M. Consumer confusion triggers crackdown by states on discount health plans. *Kaiser Health News*, April 28, 2010.

22. Blue Cross investigation is expanded. *Baltimore Sun*, March 29, 2011.

23. Galewitz, P. Hospitals adopt drug industry sales strategy. *Kaiser Health News*, December 13, 2011.

24. Meier, B. Medical experts dispute a hospital's claims on heart device data. *New York Times*, April 21, 2011.

25. Carreyrou, J, McGinty, T, Millman, J. In small California hospitals, the marketing of back surgery. *Wall Street Journal*, February 9, 2012: A1.

26. Carreyrou, J. Home-health firms blasted. *Wall Street Journal*, October 3, 2011: B1.

27. Schneiderman, L. The media and the medical market. *Cambridge Quarterly of Health Care.* Spring, 2007.

28. Rosenberg, M. Fourteen years of deceptive television drug advertising.

OpEdNews.com. Reprinted by Public Citizen's Health Research Group in *Health Letter* 27 (5): 7,9, 2011.

29. Willman, D. How a new policy led to seven deadly drugs. *Los Angeles Times,* December 20, 2000.

30. Smith, R. Medical journals are an extension of the marketing arm of pharmaceutical companies. *PLoS Medicine* 2 (5): e138, 2005.

31. Light, DW. *The Risks of Prescription Drugs.* New York. Columbia University Press And Social Science Research Council, 2010: p. 86.

32. Barrett, D, Martin, TW. Pharmacies swept into drug wars. *Wall Street Journal,* February 15, 2012: B1.

33. Ornstein, C, Weber, T. How does the medical industry influence patient care? *ProPublica* and *USA Today,* and reprinted by Public Citizen's Health Research Group in *Health Letter* 27 (6): 7-9, 2011.

34. Al-Khatib, SM, Hellcamp, A, Curtis, J et al. Non-evidence-based ICD implantations in the United States. *JAMA* 305 (1): 43-9, 2011.

35. Meier, B. Hip implants U.S. rejected sold overseas. *New York Times*, February 15, 2012: A1.

36. Elliott, C. Useless studies, real harm. Op-Ed. *New York Times*, July 29, 2011.

37. Krumholz, SD, Egilman, DS, Ross, JS. Study of Neurontin: titrate to effect, profile of safety (STEPS) trial. *Arch Intern Med* 171 (12): 1100-07, 2011.

CHAPTER 10

Bill Your Lies Correctly: How Deregulated Markets Perpetuate Health Care Fraud

"Health care fraud remains uncontrolled, and mostly invisible. For Americans, this problem represents one of the most massive and persistent fiscal control failures in their history. Many who work the system, or feed off it, like it so. For those who profit from it, health care fraud is not seen as a problem, but as an enormously lucrative enterprise, worth defending vigorously."

—Malcolm K. Sparrow, leading authority on fraud and fraud control, professor of practice of public management at Harvard University's John F. Kennedy School of Government, and author of *License to Steal, How Fraud Bleeds America's Health Care System.*[1]

In the largest Medicare fraud bust ever in five different states, FBI raids in July 2010 resulted in the arrest of 36 people, including several physicians and nurses, charged with scams totaling more than $250 million. The scams involved health professionals, clinic owners, patients, and patient recruiters. In one instance, a Brooklyn, NY facility paid patients, which unbeknownst to them included undercover agents, in exchange for using their Medicare numbers and a bonus fee for recruiting new patients. Bogus claims for physical therapy services totaling $72 million were submitted before the operation was shut down. In a separate Brooklyn case, six patients were indicted for shopping their Medicare numbers to various clinics, resulting in submission of more than 3,700 false claims for one woman over six years.[2]

The above case is one example of criminal fraud that was actually discovered and dealt with by regulators, but that success story is unfortunately not as common as it should be. Fraud in U.S health care is rampant, under-recognized, and big business.

The National Health Care Anti-Fraud Association (NHCAA), established in 1985, gives us some idea of just how big the problem is. In its 2010 white paper *Combating Health Care Fraud in a Post-Reform World: Seven Guiding Principles for Policymakers,* the NHCAA tells us that precise numbers are unknown, but the Federal Bureau of Investigation (FBI) estimates that it consumes somewhere between 3 and 10 percent of the annual health care dollar. In 2008, for example, the 10 percent level would have been $234 billion, roughly the equivalent of the GDP of countries the size of Columbia and Finland.[3] This is hardly surprising in view of the slippery slope of degrading "ethics" we saw in the last chapter as deregulated markets pursue profits above all else.

This chapter takes on three goals: (1) to provide a brief overall perspective on health care fraud; (2) to assess how pervasive it is? ; and (3) to ask how we are doing in controlling this problem?

AN OVERALL PERSPECTIVE

It would be easy to think, as so many do, that because some degree of health care fraud has always been with us, what's the big deal now? But that view would miss the boat entirely, even as it allows a huge and lucrative "industry" to stay in place. As you will soon see, health care fraud is a serious national problem that steals large sums from patients, their families, employers and taxpayers. Much of it is white-collar crime, often so invisible as to avoid detection. And when discovered, punishments tend to be light.

For starters, these definitions by Health Plus, an anti-fraud organization in New York City and Nassau County, help to lay out the overall parameters of health care fraud and distinguish it from abuse:[4]

Fraud: intentional deception or misrepresentation for the purpose of unauthorized gain to the perpetrator, including any act constituting fraud under federal or state law, committed by a managed care organization, contractor, subcontractor, provider, beneficiary or enrollee, or other persons.

Abuse: any practice that is inconsistent with sound fiscal, business, or medical practices that results in unnecessary cost to payers, or in reimbursement for services that are not medically necessary or that fail to meet professionally recognized standards for health care.

We turn to Professor Malcolm Sparrow, quoted above, for further insight into this critical problem of health care fraud. Arguably the leading expert in the country on detection and control of fraud, he has some ten years of experience as a detective, was a former detective chief inspector with the British police service, holds a Ph.D. in mathematics, and teaches regulatory and enforcement policy and operational risk control at Harvard. His book *License to Steal: How Fraud Bleeds America's Health Care System*, first published in 1996 and updated in 2000, remains a classic in the field.

In it he details a myriad of health care scams involving virtually all parts of the health care system, including physicians, dentists, other health care professionals, insurers, hospitals, clinical laboratories, home health care providers, insurers, Medicare contractors, billing specialists, our largest corporations, organized crime, and others.

Fraud schemes may involve a countless number of methods, a few of which are illustrated by these examples:

Columbia/HCA, the largest hospital chain in the country:[5]
- Disguised claims for expenses unrelated to patient care.
- Misrepresented operating expenses.
- Misidentified capitol costs for projects.
- Banning employees and consultants from disclosing existence of second set of cost reports.
- False claims for unnecessary services, those not ordered by physicians, or those never received by patients.
- Double billing for some therapies.

Managed Care Insurance Plans:[6]
- Withholding payments to providers, provider networks, or subcontractors.
- Destruction of claims.
- Embezzlement of capitation funds paid by the state.
- Fraudulent related-party transactions.
- Collusive bid-rigging between plans.

- "Bust-outs" (money received, not paid out to vendors, then entrepreneur files for bankruptcy or disappears).
- Falsification of records.
- Kickbacks to primary care physicians for referring sicker patients to "out of network" specialists.
- Denial of treatment.
- Charging exorbitant "administrative fees" while short-changing patient care.

Medicare Contractors (fiscal intermediaries), mostly BlueCross/ BlueShield):[7,8]
- Falsified documents
- Falsified administrative costs and number of claims processed.
- Payment of private insurance claims with Medicare funds.
- Obstruction of federal audits.
- Concealment of poor performance.

Most health care fraud involves false claims of one kind or another. Perpetrators of fraud become expert at falsifying claims of "patients" and "doctors," who may or not be alive! When their claims appear to follow all the rules for processing, they are typically paid without question by payers, since the health care industry has minimal routine procedures in place to determine if claims as presented are actually true. Criminals hold an unfair advantage over payers, as Malcolm Sparrow observes:

"The health industry's controls are weakest with respect to out-right criminal fraud. By contrast the industry's controls perform reasonably well in managing the grey and more ambiguous issues-such as questions about medical orthodoxy, pricing, and the limits of policy coverage. But criminals, who are intent on stealing as much as they can as fast as possible, and who are prepared to fabricate diagnoses, treatments, even entire medical episodes, have a relatively easy time breaking through all the industry's defenses. The criminals' advantage is that they are willing to lie. And provided they learn to submit their bills correctly, they remain free to lie. The rule for criminals is simple: if you want to steal from Medicare or Medicaid, or any other health care insurance program, learn to *bill your lies correctly*. Then, for the most part, your claims will be paid in full and on time, without a hiccup, by a computer, and with no human involvement at all."[9]

HEALTH CARE FRAUD: A FEW BAD APPLES OR A WIDESPREAD EPIDEMIC?

The prevalence of health care fraud boggles the mind—estimates of fraud losses range from 3 to 14 percent. If we assume that it is 10 percent, that would be some 100 times the benchmark for "acceptable business risk" set by the credit care industry! Yet measures allocated to health care fraud detection and control represent only about 0.1 percent of health program payouts.[10]

The scope and range of fraud makes the case for much more regulation with teeth. Here are several of many examples that indicate how pervasive and embedded fraud is in the health care marketplace. They also illustrate the challenges to detection and control of this widespread problem that sucks large sums of money from patients, families and taxpayers alike.

- Bass Orthopedic, a fictitious company used as a front with nothing more than two rented mailboxes and a phone number, was paid $2.1 million by Medicare over a six-month period in 1993-4. Phony billings listed the names of physicians and hundreds of patients, none of whom had heard of the company. No services were ever provided. Most of the money disappeared along with the owner by the time authorities were alerted.[11]
- In 1999, 13 podiatrists and 5 assistants were charged for Medicare fraud in New York City, where they set up a front, "Citywide Footcare" offering free foot", exams to elderly and minority residents in low-income neighborhoods. They were charged with fraud after billing Medicare for about $30 million between 1996 and 1998 for mostly fraudulent services.[12]
- In August 2011, a Los Angeles jury convicted a local pastor and his wife of fraudulently billing $14.2 million to Medicare. They had recruited parishioners to help run bogus durable medical equipment companies, then spent the receipts on expensive cars and other luxuries.[13]

- National Medical Enterprises (NME), as owners of one of the country's largest psychiatric hospital chains, pleaded guilty in 1994 for paying kickbacks and bribes for patient referrals. Community and church workers were recruited to refer patients for psychiatric care, some of whom were placed in locked wards. NME paid the government $362.7 million to settle the matter, the largest such settlement at the time.[14]
- A 1999 GAO report reviewed seven criminal health care fraud scams by organized crime involving more than 160 sham medical entities. They were mostly on-paper, making extensive use of patient brokering, rent-a-patient schemes, recruiters and runners, drop boxes, bogus corporations, and phony corporate bank accounts. Fraudulent claims ranged from $795,000 to more than $120 million.[15]
- Another GAO report in 1999 showed that more than $275 million was paid to the government in criminal fines and civil settlements by Blue Cross/Blue Shield Medicare intermediaries in five states for deceptive and improper practices that went undiscovered for years since the Health Care Financing Administration (HCFA) relied so much on information submitted by the carriers without verification.[16]

In an extensive 2008 article in *Social Research*, Sparrow identified these structural features of U.S. health care that make fraud an attractive business for criminals:

- Fee-for-service reimbursement.
- Private sector involvement.
- Highly automated claims-processing systems.
- Processing accuracy emphasized over verification.
- Postpayment audits focus on medical appropriateness, not truthfulness.[17]

The usual approach to fraud detection and control has been inadequate, too trusting, and based on a "pay and chase" strategy— payments are made first, then authorities try to run down fraud perpetrators after losses occur.

Beyond financial losses to the government, taxpayers, insurers, and employers, the human dimension of health care fraud has insidious impacts on patients, including being subjected to unnecessary, potentially harmful procedures; falsification of their medical records; becoming ineligible for future employment or insurance coverage; and being told in the future that his or her insurance coverage has reached the maximum lifetime cap on benefits.[18, 19]

In view of this serious and typically visible threat, the NHCAA has this to say:

"Given the impact on individual victims—both direct and indirect—it is clear that health care fraud is not a "victimless crime." The seriousness of the threat and the enormity of the challenge posed by health care fraud cannot be overstated."[20]

The FBI has bluntly summarized the problem this way:

"[Health care fraud] increases healthcare costs for everyone. It is as dangerous as identity theft. Fraud has left many thousands of people injured. Participation in health care fraud is a crime. Keeping America's health system free from fraud requires active participation from each of us."[21]

HOW GOES THE WAR ON HEALTH CARE FRAUD?

Serious efforts have been made by the government to rein in all this health care fraud. The Clinton Administration "declared war" on health care fraud and abuse in 1993. Then Attorney General Janet Reno called health care fraud the Department of Justice's number two priority—second only to violent crime. Two years later, a five-state demonstration project, "Operation Restore Trust," was started to test federal-state partnerships combating Medicare and Medicaid fraud, particularly in home health care, nursing homes, and durable medical equipment. Later legislation included the Health Insurance Portability and Accountability Act of 1996 (HIPPA) (which established a Health Care Fraud and Abuse Control Program (HCFAC) and a Medicare Integrity Program) and the Balanced Budget Act of 1997 (BBA) (which added new provisions, such as empowering the secretary of HHS to refuse or terminate provider agreements based on a felony, and setting penalties for hospitals that contract with excluded providers).[22] The Office of Inspector General (OIG) measured overpayment rates for Medicare from 1996 to 2002, while tracking of the return rate ratios per dollar spent on the program. It had average return rates of about 17 to 1. After several years, the Clinton administration announced progress in cutting these rates almost in half, but this turned out to be premature optimism.[23]

So how are we doing in the war on health care fraud? We are winning to the limited extent that fraud has been detected and prosecuted. But it has become clear that we have dealt with only the tip of the iceberg. Anti-fraud efforts are more intense, and progress is being made. These few examples describe some of the successes in detection and prosecution of health care fraud in recent years. Note how big these players are—this level of fraud is not accidental—it is fully intentional, and shows how far we still have to go to get a handle on the problem.

Insurers
- In 2010, regulators charged the American Trade Association, based in Tennessee, and its affiliates with selling fake health insurance to at least 26,000 households in all 50 states. They took in more than $14 million in premiums over 16 months. Some small claims were paid to appear legitimate, but big claims for sicker patients were left unpaid. A Tennessee judge ordered the liquidation of the companies, whose unpaid claims were estimated at more than $5 million.[24]

Hospitals
- HCA, the largest investor-owned hospital chain in the country, has paid $1.7 billion to the federal government, including a $900 million settlement in 2000 for Medicare payment manipulation, kickbacks, bill coding fraud and padding.[25]

Drug industry
- In 2009, Pfizer paid $2.3 billion to the federal government, a record at the time, including $1.3 billion under the False Claims Act and $1.3 billion as a criminal fine for paying kickbacks to physicians and other criminal offenses.[26]
- In November 2011, GlaxoSmithKline (GSK), the world's

fourth largest pharmaceutical company, announced a $3 billion settlement with the federal government—a new record—promoting several drug for unapproved uses, including paying kickbacks to physician prescribers; that amount is still way below its profits of $5 billion on $43 billion of sales in just the previous year.[27] Over the last 20 years, Public Citizen has found that GSK has paid fines of $4.5 billion, more than any other drug company, for various illegal activities.[28]

- After a seven-year investigation, Merck agreed to pay $950 million in November 2011, and plead guilty to settle a criminal misdemeanor charge that it had illegally promoted Vioxx for an unapproved use (treatment of pain of rheumatoid arthritis) and deceived the government about its safety after it had been shown to increase the risks of heart attacks and strokes.[29]

Supplement industry

- In 2008, Steven Warshak, founder and CEO of Berkeley Premium Nutraceuticals in Cincinnati, Ohio, and manufacturer of Enzyte, was found guilty on 93 counts of conspiracy, fraud and money laundering. Enzyte was widely advertised on national television, featuring "Smilin' Bob," as a natural male enhancement tablet without any testing or scientific basis. Warshak was sentenced to 25 years in prison, reduced to 10 years in 2011.[30]

Hospices

- Some of the country's largest hospice companies are paying multimillion-dollar settlements for fraud claims and facing multiple investigations by federal and state law enforcement agencies. In the interest of maximizing income, they are cherry-picking, longer-surviving patients, such as those with Alzheimer's dementia, over patients likely to have shorter stays, such as those with cancer. A recent report by the Inspector General of HHS has found that Medicare is paying for-profit hospices 29 percent more per beneficiary than not-for-profit hospices.[31]
- At the start of 2012, a whistleblower lawsuit led to federal charges against AseraCare, an Arkansas-based hospice company operating in 19 states. The company is charged with pressuring its employees to enroll patients into hospice who weren't dying,

resisting their discharge when they didn't get worse, and gaming hospice and nursing home stays in order to maximize Medicare reimbursement.[32]

The Odds Still Favor the Crooks

There is no question that health care fraud is being taken more seriously by government, especially in the last 15 years. Significant progress has been made. In FY 2010, the Department of Justice opened more than 1,100 new criminal health care fraud investigations involving 2,095 potential defendants Federal prosecutors had nearly 1,800 health care fraud criminal investigations pending. A total of 726 defendants were convicted for health care fraud-related crimes during the year. Also in FY 2010, HHS's Office of Inspector General (OIG) excluded 3,340 individuals and entities, based on criminal convictions for crimes related to Medicare and Medicaid (894) or to other health care programs (247), or as a result of licensure revocations (1,582). In addition, OIG issued many audits and evaluations with recommendations for steps that could correct program vulnerabilities. In all, the federal government recovered about $2.5 billion in health care fraud judgments and settlements in that year.[33]

A 2006 OIG report found that some $27 million in Medicaid payments had been made in 10 states for patient care services that were supposedly delivered *after* their deaths. In 2008, the Senate Permanent Subcommittee on Investigations revealed that between $60 million and $92 million had been paid from 2000 to 2007 for medical services or equipment that had been ordered or prescribed by dead doctors. Some of the doctors had been dead for more than 10 years at the time they supposedly ordered or prescribed treatments![34]

Based on lessons learned by hard experience in recent years, regulators are changing their approach in some ways. Since CEOs of drug and medical device makers, nursing home chains and other firms often get off free after settlements are made, federal regulators are starting to target CEOs. In the future, in addition to fines paid by companies, their executives may face criminal charges even if they weren't aware of the fraudulent scheme but could have stopped it had they known.[35] Regulators are also gaining access to billing data as they are submitted, allowing them to get a jump on the older method of "pay and chase."[36]

Despite all this progress, the crooks are still in the driver's seat. In fact, federal authorities tell us that organized crime is starting to shift from drugs to health care fraud, finding it more lucrative and safer. Regulators' budgets are still under-funded, and their staffs overextended. Automated billing and payments systems can still be readily exploited by fraud perpetrators. In fact, if a bill is submitted to Medicare for a dead patient or doctor, the perpetrator just receives a rejection letter that allows him to "clean up" his data base by eliminating that name![37] In the case of physicians caught up in marketing fraud or kickbacks with drug and medical device companies, they also get off easy. According to ProPublica, none of the more than 75 physicians named as participants in fraud by drug and medical device makers since 2008 were sanctioned, despite allegations of fraud or practices that put their patients at risk.[38] The latest OIG report found that many Medicare contractors have been relatively inactive and ineffective in detecting fraud; one contractor referred only two cases of potential fraud to Medicare officials between 2005 and 2008, while another reported none.[39]

The experienced observations and advice of Professor Sparrow indicate the daunting task ahead to develop a more structured approach to detection and fraud control:

"It is no longer sensible to disburse public funds, on trust, through electronic systems. The commensurate risks are enormous, and seriously underestimated. . . Absent some fundamental reassessment of electronic payment systems, we are doomed to continue dealing with serious fraud threats on a case-by-case rather than on a structural basis. Happily, each case detected provides some (false) assurance because it was, after all, *detected*. And each successive scandal offers an opportunity for officials to proclaim, once again, their 'zero-tolerance' for fraud in vital public programs."[40]

Ralph Nader encapsulates the economic and political challenges of health care fraud in this way:

"All in all, the health care industry is replete with rackets that neither honest practitioners or regulators find worrisome enough to effectively challenge. The perverse economic incentives in this industry range from third party payments to third party procedures. Add paid-off members of Congress who starve enforcement budgets and the enormous profits that come from that tired triad 'waste, fraud and abuse' and you have a massive problem needing a massive solution."[41]

Concerning the future, several conclusions stand out: Health care fraud remains a critical and mostly invisible problem. It is widespread and deeply embedded throughout our market-based system. The multi-payer insurance industry is part of the problem. Health care markets will need to be more tightly regulated if we are to get a handle on this problem. A larger role of government will be required to provide adequate checks and balances against health care fraud in both the private and public sectors. We need more effective approaches to detect and control it, together with better funding for state and federal agencies to pursue it. A massive reform effort will be required to root out fraud, including reform of our financing and payment systems, administrative simplification, and bringing more accountability to this runaway, freewheeling, profit-driven health care marketplace. We will return to that challenge in Chapter 12.

References

1. Sparrow, MK. *License to Steal: How Fraud Bleeds America's Health Care System*. Boulder, CO. Westview Press, 2000, p. xvii.
2. Quijano, E. Feds bust 36 for alleged Medicare scams. CBS News, July 17, 2010.
3. NHCAA. *Combating Health Care Fraud in a Post-Reform World: Seven Guiding Principles for Policymakers*. National Health Care Anti-Fraud Association. Washington, D.C. October 6, 2010.
4. Condensed from definitions developed by Health Plus, an anti-fraud organization in New York City and Nassau County (as stated in NYCRR Title 10, Chapter II, Part 98). (Htpp://www.healthplus-ny.org/en/5945_ENG_HTML.html)
5. Ibid # 1: 7-12.
6. Ibid # 1: 106-8.
7. Hallam, K, Taylor, M. Fraud fighters gain muscle. *Modern Healthcare*, August 16, 1999.

8. General Accounting Office. Medicare Improprieties by Contractors Compromised Medicare Program Integrity. GAO/OSI-99-7, July 14, 1999.
9. Sparrow, MK. Testimony before Senate Committee on the Judiciary: Subcommittee on Crime and Drugs. *Criminal Prosecution as a Deterrent to Health Care Fraud.* May 20, 2009.
10. Ibid # 9.
11. Dubocq, T. Phantom firms bleed Medicare: cost of fraud in Florida is estimated at $1 billion. *Miami Herald*, August 14, 1994: A1.
12. Smith, GB. Foot docs charged in $30 million Medicare scam. *Daily News* (New York), September 9, 1999, p. 5.
13. Sparrow, MK. An e-ripoff of the U.S. Disbursing public funds electronically sets up the federal government to be victimized by massive fraud. *Los Angeles Times* on line, August 21, 2011.
14. Myerson, AR. Hospital chain sets guilty plea: Kickbacks, bribes paid for referrals. *New York Times*, June 29, 1994: C1 (N) and D1 (L).
15. General Accounting Office. Office of Special Investigations, Washington, D.C. GAO/OSI-00-1R, October 5, 1999.
16. General Accounting Office. Medicare improprieties by contractors compromised Medicare program integrity. Washington, D.C. GAO/OSI-99-7, July 14, 1999.
17. .Sparrow, MK. Fraud in the .S. healthcare system: Exposing the vulnerabilities of automated payments systems. *Social Research* 75 (4): 1151-80, 2008.
18. Menn, J. ID theft infects medical records. *Los Angeles Times*, September 25, 2006: A1.
19. Konrad, W. Medical problems could include identity theft. *New York Times*, June 12, 2009.
20. Ibid # 3: p. 6.
21. FBI. Financial Crimes Report to the Public. FY 2006.
22. Ibid # 1: 56-9.
23. Ibid # 9: 4.
24. Lyon, L. Insurance that really isn't. *U.S. News & World Report*, August 2010, p. 40.
25. Socken, DR. *International Whistleblower Archive.* (www.whistleblowing.us)
26. Ibid # 25.
27. Public Citizen. Outrage of the Month! For Big PhRMA, crime pays. *Health Letter* 27 (11): 10, 2011.
28. Public Citizen. Rapidly increasing criminal and civil monetary penalties against the pharmaceutical industry: 1991 to 2010. (www.citizen.org/hrg1924)
29. Loftus, P, Kendall, B. Merck to pay $950 million Vioxx settlement. *Wall Street Journal*, November 23, 2011: B3.
30. Enzyte. Wikipedia, accessed January 3, 2012 (htpp://en.wikipedia.org/wiki/Enzyte)
31. Kennedy, K. Medicare costs for hospice up 70 percent. *USA Today*, August 7, 2011.
32. Rau, J. Lawsuit accuses company of fraudulently cycling patients through

nursing homes, hospice care. *Kaiser Health News*, January 4, 2012.

33. Annual Report for Fiscal Year 2010. Department of Health and Human Services and Department of Justice. Health Care Fraud and Abuse Control Program. Washington, D.C. January 2011, pp. 1-2.

34. Ibid # 9: 6.

35. Alonzo-Zaldivar, R. Feds now target execs, not just companies, in health frauds. Associated Press, May 31, 2011.

36. Ibid # 2.

37. Ibid # 31.

38. Weber, T, Ornstein, C. Doctors avoid penalties in suits against medical firms. *The Washington Post* and *ProPublica,* as reprinted by Public Citizen in *Health Letter* 27 (10): 6, 2011.

39. Kennedy, K. Medicare fraud: problems persist with contractors paid millions to ferret out bogus bills. *HuffPost Business,* November 14, 2011.

40. Ibid # 13.

41. Nader, R. In the public interest. Follow the hospital bills. *The Progressive Populist* 18 (4): 19, March 1, 2012.

PART III

BEYOND MARKET FAILURE, WHAT CAN WE EXPECT?

"The big idea is what matters in determining mortality and health in a society is less the overall wealth of that society and more how evenly wealth is distributed. The more equally wealth is distributed the better the health of that society."

—Editor's choice. 'The Big Idea'. *British Medical Journal* 312 (7037); 1996.

"When we take into view the mutual happiness and united interests of the states of America, and consider the important consequences to arise from a strict attention of each, and of all, to every thing which is just, reasonable and honourable; or the evils that will follow from an inattention to those principles; there cannot, and ought not, to remain a doubt, but that the governing rule of *right* and mutual good must in all public cases finally preside."

—Thomas Paine, 1780 (Thomas Paine, *Collected Writings*. Public Good. Foner, E. (Ed). New York. The Library of America, 1995, p. 254)

CHAPTER 11

Will Deregulated Markets Bankrupt U.S. Health Care?

"It is said that a near-death experience forces one to reevaluate priorities and values. The global economy has just had a near-death experience. The crisis exposed not only flaws in the prevailing economic model but also flaws in our society. Too many people had taken advantage of others. A sense of trust had been broken."[1]

—Joseph E. Stiglitz, Ph.D., author of *Freefall: America, Free Markets, and the Sinking of the World Economy*

"It is no measure of health to be well adjusted to a profoundly sick society."

—Jiddu Krishnamurti (1895-1986), world-renowned writer, speaker and philosopher

Over the last eight chapters we have seen the "magic" of health care markets as they really work, not as their advocates tell us they work. We have seen how the supply side runs the health care "system," largely for its own interests and often at odds with the needs of patients, families and the public interest. Continued escalation of uncontrolled health care costs is the Achilles heel of the entire system, which is not sustainable in its present form. Having completed a tour of the impacts of the market-based system on patients and families, it is not an outlandish question to ask whether this enormous medical-industrial-complex, without fundamental course changes, may actually bankrupt itself.

Our system features intense competition—between various providers against each other and against insurers, between drug companies and other industries, and among insurers for market share, while all players lobby the government for industry-friendly laissez faire policies and maximal reimbursement from public programs. The problem is that patients and taxpayers, who pay for this system, have little say over this competition. Others decide what services are needed and how much they will cost. Patients, far from exerting influence with choice, just watch as their financial burden keeps increasing. In many parts of the economy, choices made by buyers can exercise restraint on sellers, but not here in health care. The supply side in health care competes amongst themselves for the patients' and taxpayers' money while patients and voters have little control over the outcome.

This chapter asks these questions: (1) how can we summarize the adverse impacts of our market-based system on patient care and our social cohesion as a society?; (2) after going through this latest iteration of health care reform, can the Affordable Care Act (ACA) save us?; and (3) how do all the changes in health care fit into the larger context of socioeconomic changes that have occurred over the last four decades or so?

THE DOWNSIDES OF DEREGULATED MARKETS IN U.S. HEALTH CARE

Given the trends we have reviewed, including the widening gap between the wealthy, working Americans and the poor, here is a stark picture of our current predicament:

1. Uncontrolled Inflation of Health Care Costs.
- U.S. health care expenditures were $2.6 trillion in 2010, $8,402 per capita, and 17.9 percent of GDP[2]; they are projected to grow by 5.8 percent each year to $4.6 trillion in 2020, reaching $13,709 per capita and 19.8 percent of GDP.[3]
- The total cost of health care for a family of four covered by a preferred provider plan (PPO) in 2011 was $19,393, with employees paying more than 40 percent of those costs.[4]
- A recent analysis by the Commonwealth Fund found that premiums for family health insurance increased by an average

of 50 percent across all 50 states between 2003 and 2010, and are projected to reach almost $24,000 by 2020.[5]

2. *Decreased Ability to Pay for Health Care.*

- High unemployment, continued loss and erosion of health insurance coverage, and increasing cost-sharing have all contributed to many Americans delaying or forgoing care altogether since the start of this recession.[6]
- A December 2010 Health Tracking Poll by the Kaiser Family Foundation found that 54 percent of Americans reported delaying necessary care that year, with 85 percent of the uninsured delaying care due to costs and 48 percent having trouble paying their medical bills.[7]
- Two million patients with cancer are now forgoing necessary care every year because of costs that they can't afford to pay.[8]
- One half of workers with health insurance covered by small employers have an annual deductible of single coverage of $1,000 or more.[9]
- High costs are forcing an increasing number of patients to pay their health care bills with "medical credit cards. But issuers are charging exorbitant rates (e.g. GE's CareCredit card has rates as high as 26.99 percent).[10]

3. *Declining Access to Necessary Health Care.*

- A 2011 GAO report found that less than one half of U.S. physicians are willing to accept children with Medicaid and CHIP as new patients, and more than four-fifths had difficulty in referring these patients to specialty consultants.[11]
- A 2011 national study found that two-thirds of children with Medicaid were denied an appointment at a physician's office compared to just 11 percent with private coverage.[12]
- In 2011, about 80,000 patients left ERs without treatment in hospitals owned by HCA, the country's largest for-profit hospital chain, after they were told that they would have to pay $150 because they did not have a true emergency. There is now a growing trend for many U.S. hospitals to charge uninsured patients up to $350 before they can receive treatment in ERs.[13] While hospitals are required by law to at least screen patients in their ERs, they are not required to render treatment for non-

emergency conditions. The definition of an emergency has now become controversial (e.g. a severe ankle sprain is not considered an emergency in Washington State hospitals, while an ankle fracture is).[14]

- Recent draconian cuts in Medicaid have decimated safety net coverage for many Americans. For example, Medi-Cal—as the source of medical care for one in five Californians, requires co-payments of $50 for an ER visit and $100 per day in the hospital, limits enrollees to just seven physician office visits per year, and will pay physicians only $11 per patient visit.[15] Another example—starting in 2012, Hawaii plans to cut Medicaid coverage to just 10 days a year in the hospital.[16]

- A recent Harvard study found that access to psychiatric care in the greater Boston area is severely limited—only 12 percent of 64 facilities listed by Blue Cross Blue Shield of Massachusetts's PPO offered appointments for urgent care, even after they had been seen in an ER for depression and discharged with instructions to get a psychiatric appointment within two weeks.[17]

- Even as we have made impressive gains in treating the disease, nearly three out of four people in this country with HIV do not have access to necessary care. The result has massive public health consequences: they have not achieved viral suppression and can still infect others.[18]

- Inadequate access to dental care is a serious national problem. Medicare does not cover routine dental care or most dental procedures, including tooth extractions. Ten states offer *no* Medicaid coverage for dental services; the others offer a hodgepodge of services with mostly inadequate Medicaid coverage. As a result, many patients seek care in ERs for dental pain. Many of these problems are serious and even life-threatening without dental and medical treatment, especially for patients with accompanying medical illnesses. We saw one such example in Chapter 2 (p.37). Not only is dental care in ERs more expensive than outpatient dental care, it is also often inadequate, especially since dental extractions are not part of emergency physicians' armamentarium.[19]

4. A Massive Private Bureaucracy Bleeding Us Dry.

- The administrative overhead of U.S. insurers is more than five times higher than that of the single-payer program in two Canadian provinces.[20]

- A private health insurance industry of some 1,300 private insurers, each with the goal of maximizing income by selecting out the healthiest enrollees and shifting the most expensive patients to public programs. A 2012 report from the Agency for Healthcare Research and Quality found that only 5 percent of people account for one-half of national health care spending, with just one percent of the non-institutionalized population accounting for 21.8 percent of total spending.[21] These are the patients that private insurers avoid at all costs!

- According to the medical director of the Chicago-based Blue Cross Blue Shield Association, there are about 17,000 different health insurance plan designs in that area.[22]

5. Increased Tiering of Care.

- Tiering of health plans is now commonplace. Employers seek out lower premiums from insurers, typically for care by the least expensive physicians and hospitals (Tier 1). Primary care physicians often end up in different tiers for different health plans. Patients find it almost impossible to figure out their best value in choosing among tiers. As one example in Massachusetts, Sarah Bechta, M.D., who spent six to eight hours assessing choices for her family among plans, ended up saying: "There's no way my pediatrician can be tier 1 for one insurer and tier 3 [the most expensive] for another, it just makes no sense."[23]

- The 90 million individuals covered by one or another chronically under-funded public programs, such as Medicaid and SCHIP, have difficulty finding physicians to see them, and when seen, are seen only briefly, often for less than 10 minutes.[24]

- When seen in ERs, uninsured and Medicaid patients receive fewer imaging tests than their insured counterparts, and when they do receive such tests, they are of lower clinical value.[25]

- Despite their tax breaks and wealth, children's hospitals provide on average only about two percent of their budgets on free medical care; some of the largest elite hospitals spend less than one percent on charity care.[26]

6. *Decreased Quality and Worse Outcomes.*

- As we saw in Chapter 2 (Figure 2.2, p.39), life expectancy in the U.S. is much lower than most advanced countries around the world, despite our spending far more than any of them on health care.
- Deaths that are preventable by timely and effective care— mortality amenable to health care—is the worst in the U.S. among 16 high-income countries in the world.[27]
- Based on the latest available data from the U.S. Census Bureau and estimates by Harvard researchers of excess mortality among uninsured people, 50,000 Americans die each year for lack of health insurance—136 per day.[28]
- Compared to their not-for-profit counterparts, publicly traded, investor-owned, for-profit health plans spend less on patient care, and have worse quality of care as measured by preventive care, treatment of chronic conditions, members' access to care, and customer service.[29]
- Quality of care is lower in areas with more specialists, higher use of medical technology, and with larger amounts of unnecessary and inappropriate care.[30-32]

CAN THE AFFORDABLE CARE ACT
GET US OUT OF THIS HOLE?

Despite what we are told by its supporters, I have no confidence that this very expensive bill will effectively redress any of the above critical problems in U.S. health care. Too many political compromises have been made along the way, and one of the major barriers to real reform—*the private insurance industry itself*—was left intact and even further subsidized by the government. Private health care markets across the entire medical-industrial-complex were largely left to their own devices, without price controls and with considerable latitude to game the new system. The government boxed itself in politically, fearing that if it got too tough on private insurers that they would give up coverage, increase the number of uninsured and further exacerbate the access problem. It bowed to the political power and money of corporate stakeholders with many of its claimed regulatory mechanisms more posturing than likely to be effective in reaching its three major goals—assuring access, containing costs, and increasing the quality of care.

As described my 2010 book *Hijacked: The Road to Single Payer in the Aftermath of Stolen Health Care Reform*, the ACA does have a number of potentially beneficial provisions, including these:[33]

- Extending health insurance to about 30 million more people by 2019, especially through expansion of Medicaid to 16 million lower-income Americans.
- Subsidies to help lower-income people to afford insurance.
- Providing for parents to keep their children on their policies until age 26.
- Initiation of some limited insurance reforms, such as prohibiting exclusions based on pre-existing conditions and banning of annual and lifetime limits.
- Establishing state-based high-risk pools to help the uninsured gain coverage.
- New funding for community health centers.
- Establishing government-sponsored Exchanges in every state whereby uninsured people can shop for the best value in coverage.
- Creation of a non-profit Patient-Centered Outcomes Research Institute (PCORI) tasked with assessing the relative outcomes, clinical effectiveness and appropriateness of different medical treatments.

But the 20-pound, 2,400-page bill is extremely complex and, not surprisingly since it was largely crafted to the likes of corporate stakeholders, presents them with many opportunities to keep gaming the system to their benefit. Figure 11.1 illustrates the futility of this apparatus helping patients compared to the more obvious therapy that was never on the table (Figure 11.1).

Here are just a few of the many ways in which we can expect to see the law fail to meet its intended goals:

Access to care.

There will still be 26 million uninsured in 2019 even if the ACA survives the GOP's opposition and efforts to repeal it, and even if it is fully implemented. Most of what ends up being called "insurance" will fall far short of adequate coverage. Instead of covering a defined set of benefits (as traditional Medicare does), it will provide a defined *contribution* toward the costs of care. This just ends up shifting even more costs of care to patients and their families.[34] The state-based high-risk pools serve very few patients, have to deal with adverse selection, and some states are already asking the government for more money.[35] Alaska gives us an example of the problems facing these high-risk pools—it will spend some $10 million in 2012 to cover just 50 enrollees—about $200,000 per person.[36]

FIGURE 11.1

Health Care "Reform" Drip by Drip

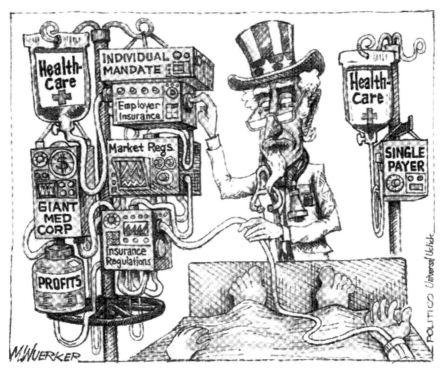

Source: Reprinted with permission from Matt Wuerker

Moreover, the supposed safety net will continue to deteriorate. The federal government has been very generous in granting waivers to states' Medicaid programs, even to the point of allowing states to eliminate hospital coverage and impose restrictions of the number of physician visits per year. More than one-half of medical practices in the U.S. are re-negotiating or eliminating low-paying commercial payer contracts as a way to deal with the economic impacts of the recession[37], many will no longer see patients on Medicare or Medicaid, and further cuts to both programs are still a political football in this election season.

Cost containment

There are no price controls for prescription drugs or mechanisms to prevent suppliers' exorbitant prices. HHS requires insurers to justify premium increases more than 10 percent a year, but lacks authority to make limits stick (it can only publicize higher rate increases). As California Insurance Commissioner Dave Jones, says: "The authority to review without the authority to reject or modify is not terribly effective."[38] Consolidation among insurers, hospitals and physician groups in accountable care organizations (ACOs) will gain market share but is not likely to contain prices and costs.[39] PCORI is prevented by law from making use of cost-effectiveness or quality-adjusted life years (QALYs) in its coverage, reimbursement and policy recommendations.[40] Over the years 2010 to 2019, the CBO has projected that health care costs will grow by $965 billion, *not* including the "doc fix" (some $200 billion for future physician reimbursement).[41] But these are only the costs borne by the government, *not* including increasing out-of-pocket costs paid by patients and their families.

Affordability of care

As costs continue to spiral upward, the numbers of unemployed and under-employed remain high, and family incomes fall increasingly short of essential needs, more people, even with insurance, will not be able to afford necessary care. Remarkably enough, despite the law's title as the Patient Protection and Affordable Care Act, we still lack any consensus as to what standard constitutes affordability. A recent study convened an expert panel of 18 experts with extensive experience in this area, but could not come to any agreement whether savings, debt, education, or single parenthood are relevant.[42] Earlier, the Commonwealth Fund had proposed this useful definition for *underinsurance—*

"People who are insured all year but report at least one of these three indicators:

1. Medical expenses amounting to 10 percent or more of income
2. Among low-income adults below 200 percent of the federal poverty level, medical expenses at or more than 5 percent of income
3. Health plan deductibles at or more than 5 percent of income."[43]

Already, a growing number of American families are paying up to 20 percent or more of their annual household income for family coverage. Even then, however, they may be underinsured for a major accident or serious illness. Given the rapid decline in defined benefit coverage, many of us are just one accident or serious medical problem away from serious personal financial hardship or bankruptcy.

Regulation of insurers

Insurers will still have wide latitude to push profits over service. They are making record profits even as patients use less health care.[44] They are already gaming the law's details to select out healthier enrollees and dump sicker people onto the government programs and Exchanges that will become operational in 2014. Medicare Advantage plans that market fitness center coverage in their plans automatically cherry pick healthier seniors with lesser health care costs.[45] While the law requires risk adjustment measures of health status, insurers will not be required to submit their data to HHS, so that there will be no way to validate their risk scores.[46] Moreover, a 2012 GAO report found that risk adjustment methods are still so crude as to be easily gamed by insurers to their advantage.[47] Insurers are also working to bend the system in their favor by seeking seats on Exchanges when they come on line in 2014.[48] And some insurers are starting private Exchanges that will compete with the government exchanges, trying to further shift the burden of sicker enrollees to the public sector.[49] The law has minimal requirements for value of policies—actuarial values of just 60 percent will become commonplace (when insurers cover just 60 percent of costs), with high-deductible plans and skinny networks of providers. Employers and insurers have a mutual interest in keeping insurance premiums "affordable", while they lobby for final essential benefits rules that are sufficiently restrictive to serve their own interests. In effect, we can anticipate an epidemic of *unaffordable underinsurance* that passes along more out-of-pocket costs to patients and their families under the illusion that progress is being made. [50]

Quality improvement.

To the extent that fee-for-service continues to dominate most health care transactions, many perverse incentives will remain with our profit-oriented market-based system. Accountable care organizations (ACOs) will have incentives to organize themselves around profits, and will be able to retain one-half of whatever moneys they gain by "savings." Quality and performance measures still are mostly concerned with process, not outcomes, which count far more. There will still be incentives among insurers to deny care, and many physicians will be pressured by their employers to restrict services. The new unproven experiments with "bundled payments" will be a work in progress for some years, with the rules still being written. Moreover, since there will still be many millions of uninsured and underinsured Americans, they will be forced to delay and forgo essential care, receive later diagnosis of serious illness, and have worse outcomes.

TWO AMERICAS: A SOCIOECONOMIC SEA CHANGE

An important part of the answer to the question posed in the title of this chapter is the financial health of those financing this mess—the consumer and the taxpayer. Their ability to keep going will run out. This is especially true if we look at the broader context and trends.

Consider how much has changed since the mid-1950s. In 1955, when Dr. Jonas Salk completed development of his polio vaccine, he was asked by Edward R. Murrow who owned the patent? Salk famously replied: "The American people, I guess. Could you patent the sun?" The March of Dimes had helped to fund its development, but declined to patent it, as did Dr. Salk. As a result, the vaccine remained cheap and freely available to everyone, leading to the eradication of polio in this country and in most other industrialized nations around the world.[51]

Given the socioeconomic tectonic shift that we have seen in America since World War II, can we imagine such a thing happening in this country today as a new technological breakthrough is made? That story illustrates the wide gulf between the America we used to be and that of today.

Noam Chomsky, distinguished linguist and political critic at the Massachusetts Institute of Technology, brings us this helpful historical perspective:

"The 1970s marked a turning point for the United States. Since the country began, it had been a developing society, not always in pretty ways, but with general progress toward industrialization and wealth. Even in dark times, the expectation was the progress would continue. . . . Now there's a sense of hopelessness, sometimes despair. This is quite new in our history. During the 1930s, working people could anticipate that the jobs would come back. Today, if you're a worker in manufacturing, with unemployment practically at Depression levels, you know that those jobs may be gone forever if current policies persist.
That change in the American outlook has evolved since the 1970s. In a reversal, several centuries of industrialization turned to de-industrialization. Of course manufacturing continued, but overseas, very profitable, though harmful to the workforce. The economy shifted to financialization. Financial institutions expanded enormously. A vicious cycle between finance and politics accelerated. Increasingly, wealth concentrated in the financial sector. Politicians, faced with the rising cost of campaigns, were driven ever deeper into the pockets of wealthy backers. And the politicians rewarded them with policies favorable to Wall Street: deregulation, tax changes, relaxation of rules for corporate governance, which intensified the vicious cycle. Collapse was inevitable. In 2008, the government once again came to the rescue of Wall Street firms presumably too big to fail, with leaders too big to go to jail. Today, for the one-tenth of 1 percent of the population who benefited most from these decades of greed and deceit, everything is fine."[52]

Wall Street is unrepentant. Citigroup, though saved by government bailouts, still targets the super rich as its growth opportunity. It has developed the Plutonomy Index, stocks in companies catering to the luxury market, in an effort to move investors in that direction,[53] while press reports continue of widespread malfeasance and greed on the "Street."

This is the America confronting us today:

- Huge and growing income gap between the 1 and 99 percent of us (see Figure 1.1, on page 24)[54]
- Increasing residential segregation of families by income that isolates the rich from ordinary Americans[55]
- Suburbanization of poverty, now not just in inner cities and isolated rural areas.[56]
- Median household incomes of typical American families has dropped for three years in a row, and is now about where it was in 1996 when adjusted for inflation.[57]
- As class lines become more rigid, social mobility is dropping—whereas 62 percent of American men and women raised in the top fifth of incomes stay in the top two-fifths, 65 percent born in the bottom fifth remain in the bottom two-fifths.[58]
- A toxic political environment, where "Super PACs" dominate disinformation campaigns and bankroll a complicit media industry.
- As our traditional social fabric becomes more tattered, comparisons with the rest of the world become even more stark; as an example, a recent report by the Bertelsmann Stiftung foundation of Germany—*Social Justice in the OECD: How Do Member States Compare* ranked the 31 countries by various metrics of basic fairness and equality; the U.S. ranked in the bottom five on five of nine metrics and in the bottom 10 on the others (including the health rating, which rated inclusiveness, quality of service, and perceived health between highest/lowest incomes).[59]

This is where unfettered, deregulated markets have taken us after more than three decades. As the nation flounders in its ongoing deep recession and the 2012 election campaign heats up, the single most important issue is over the role of government. Turning a blind eye to market failure and any concept of one America, Republicans keep arguing for smaller government (though they like to privatize whatever they can!), no new taxes, tax relief for corporations and the rich, cuts in "entitlement" programs, and repeal of the ACA. Figure 11.2 well illustrates what *not* to expect from the Tea Party, the right wing of the right!

FIGURE 11.2

Tea Party Politics

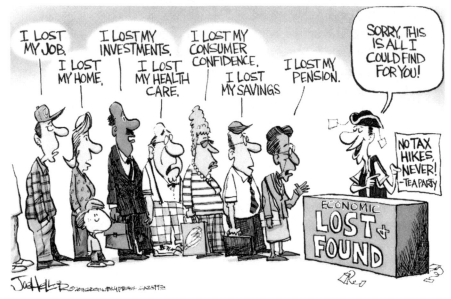

Source: Reprinted with permission from Joe Heller/*Green Bay Press-Gazette*

So health care, and its reform, are part of a much larger picture, making real reform even more daunting. Despite high technology advances, our market-based system has already shown itself to be morally and socially bankrupt, with a future risk of economic bankruptcy. Its reform in the public interest grows more urgent every day, but it will require a broad grassroots movement to roll back the sea changes over the last three decades that have corrupted our political system and weakened our democracy. The stakes are higher than ever—whether we will be one America and one people, or a bitterly divided society with a lesser future.

References

1. Stiglitz, JE. *Freefall: America, Free Markets, and the Sinking of the World Economy*. New York. W. W. Norton & Company, Inc., 2010: p. 275.
2. Radnofsky, L. Weak economy curbs health spending. *Wall Street Journal*, January 10, 2012.

3. Office of the Actuary, CMS, National Health Spending Projections through 2020. *Health Affairs*, July 28, 2011.
4. McCanne, D. The "Milliman Medical Index ($19,393) in perspective, May 12, 2011. (www.pnhp.org/blog)
5. Gold, J. Health insurance premiums soar in all 50 states. *Kaiser Health News* blog, November, 2011, 2011.
6. Martin, AB, Lassman, D, Washington, B, Catlin, A and the National Health Expenditure Accounts Team. Growth in U.S. health spending remained slow in 2010; Health share of gross domestic product was unchanged from 2009. *Health Affairs*, January 2012.
7. December Health Tracking Poll, 2010. Kaiser Family Foundation.
8. Weaver, KE, Roland, JH, Bellizzi, KM, Ariz, NM. Forgoing medical care because of cost: Assessing disparities in healthcare access among cancer survivors living in the United States. *Cancer online*, June 14, 2010.
9. Mathews, AW. Push for health-cost data. *Wall Street Journal*, October 27, 2011:B8.
10. Konrad, W. Think twice before signing up for that medical credit card. *New York Times*, November 27, 2010: B5.
11. Binder, JT. Care can be universal, cheaper. *The Charleston Gazette*, July 30, 2011.
12. Bisgaier, J, Rhodes, KV. Auditing access to specialty care for children with public insurance. *N Engl J Med* 363 (24): 2324-33, 2011.
13. Galewitz, P. Hospitals demand payment upfront from ER patients with routine problems. *Kaiser Health News*, February 20, 2012.
14. Mathews, AW. Medicaid cuts rile doctors. *Wall Street Journal*, February 25-6, 2012: A3.
15. Corcoran, D. Doctors say Medi-Cal reimbursement is too low. *San Francisco Chronicle*, August 4, 2010.
16. Galewitz, P. States are limiting Medicaid hospital coverage in search of savings. *Kaiser Health News*, October 24, 2011.
17. Boyd, JW, Linsenmeyer, A, Woolhandler, S, Himmelstein, DU, Nardin, R. The crisis in mental health care: A preliminary study of access to psychiatric care in Boston. *Ann Emerg Med* 58 (2): 218-9, 2011.
18. McKay, B. Most HIV patients lack needed care. *Wall Street Journal*, November 30, 2011: A6.
19. Bath, A. Patients visiting ER, not dentist. *USA TODAY*, January 20-22, 2012:3B.
20. Woolhandler, S, Campbell, T, Himmelstein, DU. Costs of health care administration in the United States and Canada. *N Engl J Med* 349: 768-75, 2003.
21. Rovner, J. Biggest bucks in health care are spent on a very few. *NPR News*, January 12, 2012.
22. Kagel, R. Blue crossroads: Insurance in the 21st Century. *American Medical News*, September 20, 2004.
23. Bebinger, M. "Tiered insurance confounds consumers, docs in Mass. *Kaiser Health News* January 17, 2012.

24. Garthwaite, C. The Doctor Might See You Now: The Supply Side Effects of Public Health Insurance Expansions. The National Bureau of Economic Research. *NBER Digest OnLine*, Cobober 2011.

25. Moser, JW, Applegate, KE. Imaging and insurance: Do the uninsured get less imaging in emergency departments? *J Amer College Radiology* 50 (1): 50-7, 2012.

26. Gaul, GM. Growing size and wealth of children's hospitals fueling questions about spending. *Kaiser Health News*, September 25, 2011.

27. Nolte, E, McKee, M. Variations in amenable mortality—Trends in 16 high-income countries. New York. The Commonwealth Fund, September 13, 2011.

28. Wolfe, SM. Outrage of the Month! 50 million uninsured in the U.S. equals 50,000+ avoidable deaths each year. *Health Letter* 28 (1):11, January 2012.

29. McCue, MJ, Bailit, MH. Assessing the financial health of Medicaid managed care plans and the quality of patient care they provide. New York. The Commonwealth Fund, June 15, 2011.

30. Fisher, ES, Welch, HG. Avoiding the unintended consequences of growth in medical care: How might more be worse? *JAMA* 281: 445-51, 1999.

31. Wennberg, JB, Fisher, ES, Skinner, JS. Geography and the debate over Medicare reform. *Health Affairs Web Exclusive* W-103. February 13, 2002.

32. ACP. The impending collapse of primary care medicine and its implications for the state of the nation's health care. Washington, D.C.: American College of Physicians, January 30, 2006. (http://www.acponline.org/hpp/statec06_1pdf, accessed August 10, 2006)

33. Geyman, JP. *Hijacked: The Road to Single Payer in the Aftermath of Stolen Health Care Reform*. Friday Harbor, WA. Copernicus Healthcare, 2010.

34. Orszag, P. Defined contributions define health-care future. *Bloomberg*, December 6, 2011.

35. Galewitz, P. 9 states seek help for high-risk pools. Capsules. *The KHN BLOG*, January 5, 2012.

36. Galewitz, P. Alaska to spend $22K a year for each high risk pool member. *Kaiser Health News* January 17, 2012.

37. Elliott, VS. Dropping an insurer requires care and analysis. *American Medical News*, August 9, 2010.

38. Adamy, J. Steep rises in health premiums scrutinized. *Wall Street Journal*, August 30, 2011: A5.

39. Austin, DA, Hungerford, TL. *The Market Structure of the Health Insurance Industry*. Washington, D.C. Congressional Research Service, November 17, 2009.

40. AAMC Government Relations. *Summary of Patient-Centered Outcomes Research Provisions*, March 2010.

41. CBO. The health care law. Questioning the cost of the health care overhaul. *New York Times*, April 3, 2010: A11.

42. Muennig, P, Sampat, B, Tilipman, N, Brown, LD, Glied, SA. We all want it, but we don't know what it is: Toward a standard of affordability for health insurance premiums. *J Health Politics, Policy and Law*, October 2011.

43. Schoen, C, Doty, M, Collins, SR, Holmgren, AL. Commonwealth Fund. Insured but not protected: How many adults are underinsured, the experiences of adults with inadequate coverage mirror those of their uninsured peers, especially among the chronically ill. *Health Affairs Web Exclusive*, June 14, 2005.

44. Frier, S. Insurers profit from health law they fought. *Bloomberg*, January 5, 2012.

45. Cooper, AL, Trivedi. AN. Fitness memberships and favorable selection in Medicare Advantage plans. *N Engl J Med* 366: 150-57, 2012.

46. Park, E. Allowing insurers to withhold data on enrollees' health status could undermine key part of health reform. Washington, D.C. Center on Budget and Policy Priorities. December 12, 2011.

47. GAO report on Medicare Advantage risk adjustment. Washington D.C. General Accounting Office, January 2012.

48. Carey, MA, Serafini, MW. Sweating the details: health reform supporters fret over HHS rules. *Kaiser Health News*, September 6, 2011.

49. Reichard, J. Washington health policy in review. Private exchanges may be poised to spread—with uncertain impact on health law. New York. The Commonwealth Fund, January 6, 2012.

50. Bybee, R. Health reform devolves into 'unaffordable under-insurance'. *In These Times*, December 7, 2011.

51. Smith, J. *Patenting the Sun: Polio and the Salk Vaccine*. New York. William Morrow, 1990. pp. 159,194.

52. Chomsky, N. Occupy the future. Presentation in the Howard Zinn Memorial Lecture Series held by Occupy Boston's on-site Free University. November 1, 2011.

53. Ibid # 51.

54. Ketcham, C. The new populists. *The American Prospect* 23 (1): 17, 2012.

55. Reardon, SF, Bischoff, K. Growth in the residential segregation of families by income, 1970-2009. US2010 Project, November 2011.

56. DeParle, J, Tavernise, S, Poor are still getting poorer, but downturn's punch varies, Census data show. *New York Times*, September 15, 2011: A24.

57. Dougherty, C. Income slides to 1996 levels. *Wall Street Journal*, September 14, 2011: A1.

58. DeParle, J. Harder for Americans to rise from economy's lower rungs. *New York Times*, January 5, 2012:A1.

59. Blow, CM. America's exploding pipe dream. *New York Times*, October 29, 2011: A17.

CHAPTER 12

Empowering Patients and Taxpayers: Toward Achieving Health Care That We All Want And Need

"If you ask why America is more class-bound in practice than the rest of the Western world, a large part of the reason is that our government falls down on the job of creating equal opportunity."[1]

—Paul Krugman, Ph.D. Nobel laureate in economics and author of *The Conscience of a Liberal*

"The economic and social collapse we face was presaged by a moral collapse. And our response must include a renewed reverence for moral and social imperatives that acknowledge the sanctity of the common good."[2]

—Chris Hedges, fellow at the Nation Institute, columnist for Truthdig, and author of *The World As It Is: Dispatches on the Myth of Human Progress*

Having traced developments in our health care system over the last 30-plus years and noted how they have taken place within the larger trends of socioeconomic sea changes in our society, it is now time to learn from this experience and re-focus on how we can reform the excesses of our market-based system. Preceding chapters give ample documentation of market failure in health care. We know the lessons from this grand experiment— health care markets are designed to primarily serve Wall Street and stakeholders on the supply side, not Main Street where patients and their families live. We have also shown the many ways in which the Affordable Care Act of 2010 will fall far short of needed reforms.

But all Americans, regardless of class or income, need health care of good quality readily available to us when we have an accident or get sick. This is our universal need from which we are falling so short. Whether our politics are on the right or left, we should be able to agree that we must have an accessible, efficient, fair and sustainable system that delivers health care of good quality that meets, with the least bureaucracy, our individual and population's needs.

The goals of this last chapter are (1) to discuss briefly how the health care debate can be reframed along progressive lines; (2) to note some cracks in the armor of the massive opposition in corporate America and on Wall Street to serious reform; and (3) to outline a way forward that can reorient health care markets toward the common good while continuing a robust private sector in health care.

A Way Forward: Reframing The Health Care Debate

Before considering specific frames, we need to ask some obvious and fundamental questions about what kind of a health care system we want. Recall from Chapter 1 that we posed five basic questions (p. 25), including who the health care system is for, should care be based on medical need, how should health care be financed, and how can we reform our unaccountable, unaffordable system in such a way as to make it sustainable without bankrupting us?

As is obvious from preceding chapters, the "free market" has been unable to provide the kind of system and care that we need. It is now also clear from the forgoing that we need a larger role of government to assure that health care will be available to all Americans. After some four decades of experimenting with private financing of health care, we can conclude that the experiment is over. Despite its many government subsidies (even increased by the ACA!), the private health insurance industry is terminally ill. It is a big part of our problems, and is an obstacle standing in the way of our *ever* achieving universal health care in this country.

So it is high time that we deal with these basic questions. They are still unanswered and have not even been part of the political discourse as "reform" has been debated over these many years. Amazingly enough, we have allowed corporate stakeholders in the market-based system to set policy by default through their political power, lobbying strength, control of the media, and deceptive advertising campaigns. Politicians in both major parties have been bought off along the way and are complicit with allowing market excesses to perpetuate themselves.

George Lakoff, Professor of Linguistics at the University of California Berkeley and author of *Don't Think Of An Elephant!: Know Your Values and Frame the Debate—The Essential Guide for Progressives*, gives us a good start toward reframing the debate along progressive lines. In 2007, in the heat of the 2008 election campaigns, he and his colleagues called for a larger role for government to assert its moral responsibility to empower and protect its citizens, further identifying these requirements for a just health care system:[3]

"• Everyone should have access to comprehensive, quality health care.
 • No one should be denied care for the sake of private profit.
 • You can choose your own doctor.
 • Promotion of health and well being, focusing on preventive care.
 • Costs should be progressive, that is, readily affordable to everyone, with higher costs borne by those better able to pay.
 • Access should be extremely easy, with no specific roadblocks.
 • Administration should be simple and cheap.
 • Interactions should be minimally bureaucratic and maximally human.
 • Payments should be adequate for doctors, nurses, and other health care workers.
 • When people are harmed by either the unsafe practices or negligence of health care providers, the redress should be left to the courts—with no arbitrary caps on compensatory payments."

None of these important principles surfaced in the political debates offered by either the Republicans or Democrats during that election cycle. Instead, the right followed the disinformation rhetoric of Frank Luntz, political consultant and pollster, emphasizing that single-payer means "rationing" and stoking fear of a "government takeover" vs. the claimed advantages of free markets and competition. Without a specific plan for health care, the GOP argued for a "patient-centered health care" in an open system where patients and doctors make health care decisions.[4] Meanwhile, the Democrats took an overly moderate "surrender in advance" strategy that discarded progressive policies in favor of rhetoric that would allow people to "keep your insurance if you like it," "build on our system's many strengths", and "keep insurers honest."[5]

In an earlier book in 2008, *Do Not Resuscitate: Why the Health Insurance Industry Is Dying, and How We Must Replace It,* I suggested that the entire debate over health care reform could be encapsulated by the following simple formulation:

> "Restore the promise of opportunity and security by promoting better health for our people, communities and country through enlightened health policies of fiscal prudence and fairness to all."[6]

Copernicus Healthcare, as publisher of this book, has taken a common-sense approach to these questions in calling for a paradigm shift in U.S. health care equally as "radical" as that of Nicolaus Copernicus. As we know, Copernicus was a Renaissance astronomer who departed from the "wisdom" of those in power in his time by conceiving a comprehensive heliocentric cosmology that, for the first time, displaced the Earth from the center of the universe, instead putting the sun in that center. The Copernican insight was a breakthrough that fit the facts better than the Ptolemaic version. The earth-centric vision of the universe grew too complex to be credible. That shift launched a new starting point for modern astronomy and was a landmark in the history of science.

So too in U.S. health care. Free market advocates face a growing tidal wave of facts that don't fit the obvious realities. A Copernican shift in health care puts patients and families at the center of the system instead of corporate and supply-side interests in the medical-industrial-complex, as illustrated in Figure 12.1. It goes a long way in answering the above questions and reorienting our objectives about health care by 180 degrees in these ways:[7]

- Shifting from a system based on ability to pay to one based on medical need.
- Moving from health care as a commodity for sale on a free market to a basic human need and right.
- Moving from profits driven by a business "ethic" to a largely not-for-profit system based on service.
- Moving from a dysfunctional, fragmented and exploitive private health insurance industry to a single-payer, public financing system coupled with a private delivery system.
- Moving from political and lobbyist-driven coverage policies toward those based on scientific evidence of efficacy and cost-effectiveness.
- Replacing today's unaccountable system with one that stewards limited health care resources for the benefit of all Americans.

At this writing in April 2012, in the midst of the 2012 election campaigns, our reframed principles, consistent with American values, should be:

- America is a country of people, not corporations.
- Corporations are not persons.
- It is absurd to keep paying more and getting less from health care than in other advanced countries.
- Every American is special and deserves the best health care that available resources permit.
- It doesn't make sense to bail out a failing private insurance system that depends on the government for its survival.
- Equal opportunity to necessary health care should be the American way.
- It is stupid to let our market-based system bankrupt us when there is already enough money in the system to pay for coverage of all Americans.

How we deal with these fundamentals will determine whether we are to be one nation, one people, or a divided society based on income?

FIGURE 12.1

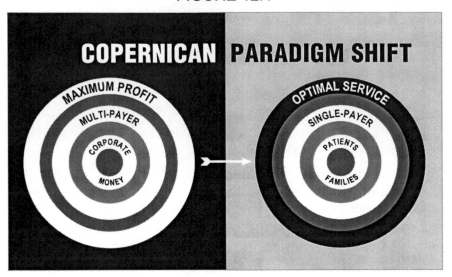

Cracks in the Armor of Conservative
Opposition to Universal Coverage

It has long been surprising to me, and to many others in this country supporting universal access to medical care for all, that conservatives keep putting up with the demonstrable flaws of our unsustainable system that clearly doesn't work for much of our population. What is easy to see, of course, is that powerful corporate interests across the entire medical-industrial-complex want to maintain their very profitable status quo. Since corporate money dominates our politics and media, this opposition is a massive barrier to health care reform.

As we saw in the last chapter, health care is just one of other big problems within our society—increasing inequality, increasing poverty, withering of the middle class, high unemployment and underemployment, for starters. We all know the list. So until we can gather enough political strength to confront the corporate kleptocracy, real health care reform remains unlikely.

But there are important chinks in the armor of this opposition, including even at the heart of American conservatism. In their landmark article in 2006, Donald Light and his philosopher colleague Paul Menzel call attention to the striking differences between conservative thought overseas and in the U.S. While they may debate some of the details, conservatives in other advanced countries give broad support to systems of universal coverage on economic, political, pragmatic and moral grounds. They recognize the advantages of universal access to essential medical care as an important factor that limits their business costs, minimizing waste, increasing worker productivity, and growing their business interests. Menzel and Light draw this conclusion:

> "It is time for American conservatives to add health care to fire and police services as minimum government services needed to enable individuals to thrive at minimal financial costs. The question for conservative leaders who deplore wasted potential, free-riding, financial waste, and inefficiency is not whether they can support universal access to needed health care. It is how they can *not* support universal access without betraying their own values."[8]

After three decades of trying one or another approach to get universal coverage in this country, it is time to recognize that we will never get there as long as it is voluntary and leaves the private health insurance industry in place. As the latest attempt, the Affordable Care Act will not get there, nor will it contain costs or resolve issues of quality and equity.

So a pivotal issue deserving our full attention is to decide, through a democratic process unhindered by corporate money (joke!), whether we go forward for this and later generations with our mostly for-profit, exploitive, duplicative multi-payer financing system or shift to a single-payer system, an improved Medicare for all, coupled with a private delivery system. In any objective comparison between the two, single-payer wins hands down—it would provide universal access to all Americans, with full choice of physicians and hospitals, reduce waste and bureaucracy, save money through global budgets and negotiated fees, and shift the dominant ethic from profits to service. It would meet the goals that conservatives espouse of greater efficiency, less waste, increased value, and more accountability. Table 12.1 summarizes the comparision.[9]

There are many reasons to hope that a powerful political groundswell is building towards a time when real health care reform is more likely, even inevitable. Here are a few of many bright spots that auger for better days ahead:

TABLE 12.1

Alternative Financing Systems and American Values

TRADITIONAL VALUE	Single-Payer	Multi-Payer
Efficiency	↑	↓
Choice	↑	↓
Affordability	↑	↓
Actuarial value	↑	↓
Fiscal responsibility	↑	↓
Equitable	↑	↓
Accountable	↑	↓
Integrity	↑	↓
Sustainable	↑	↓

• **The Occupy Movement: 99% vs. 1 %.** This is a frame that captures a lot of the anger and frustration throughout our society. As Senator Bernie Sanders (I-VT) sums up the gathering movement's strength:

> "We are now seeing from coast to coast a growing move-
> ment of ordinary Americans who understand that current
> public policy benefits the wealthiest one percent at the ex-
> pense of virtually everyone else. Every day, in their own
> states, cities and towns, they are seeing how destructive
> the right-wing agenda is for the average American. They
> know that the greed and illegal behavior of Wall Street
> caused this terrible recession and that we need real Wall
> Street reform. They know that the growing wealth and in-
> come inequality between the very rich and everyone else
> in America is immoral and economically unsustainable.
> They are standing up and saying: 'Enough is Enough! We

need real change in our country.
We need action which benefits all of us and not just the
very wealthy."[10]

The Occupy movement has already resulted in many important changes, including naming the basic problems of the 99 percent—Wall Street greed, perverse financial incentives, and the corporate takeover of our political system, charting a new way forward toward policies that will benefit the 99 percent, and rejecting the false promises of "trickle down" economics. It offers an ethic and practice of fundamental democracy and community while calling for a government that is responsive to the common good and free of corporate dominance.[11]

• *The Divestiture Movement.* Divestiture proved itself as an effective strategy for socially-constructive political action from 1985 to 1990 in South Africa. More than 200 U.S. companies cut all ties with the country, resulting in a loss of $1 billion in direct American aid. Pension funds, faith communities and others declared that they would not support injustice. As a result of people power and democracy in action, that economic pressure hastened the fall of apartheid.[12]

There is now a growing divestiture movement in this country directed at the private health insurance industry. Domini Social Investments has already disqualified most health insurers from their portfolios. The Presbyterian Church USA will vote in the summer of 2012 on an "Overture" to "implement divestment procedures as well as encourage individual Presbyterians and congregations to divest of holdings in the [publicly traded health insurance] companies." A Divestment Campaign for Health Care has been organized through the leadership of Dr. Rob Stone, emergency physician in Bloomington, IN and Director of Hoosiers for a Commonsense Health Plan, and others. Its mission is to "expose how the health insurance industry puts the need for profit above the needs of patients and to escalate public support for total removal of the private health insurance companies from our nation's healthcare."[13,14] Figure 12.2 illustrates the problem.

• *Bipartisan backlash to Paul Ryan's Medicare voucher plan.* Pushback was immediate after Ryan released his plan for Medicare—vouchers, shifting to a defined contribution (easily

FIGURE 12.2

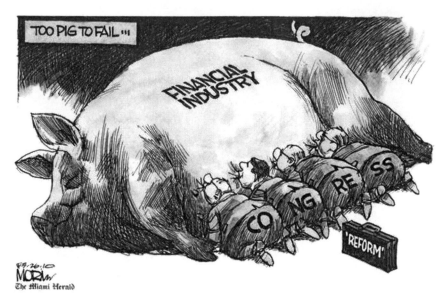

Source: Reprinted with permission from Jim Morin

reduced in the future) voucher plan from the traditional defined benefit coverage that pays about one-half of seniors' health care expenses. Democrats opposed it right out of the starting gate, but were also joined by many Republicans fearing backlash from seniors. The CBO calculated that seniors would pay much more for their health care under the "premium support" plan.[15]

- *Montana Court decision against Citizens United.* In January 2012, the Supreme Court of Montana held that the Citizens United decision does not apply to campaign finance law in Montana. It upheld the constitutionality of a 1912 voter initiative—the Corrupt Practices Act—that prohibits corporations from making contributions to state political candidates or parties.[16]
- *Wisconsin recall of Governor Scott Walker.* In January 2012, Democrats collected more than 1 million signatures to require that Governor Walker face a recall election, the first such recall in Wisconsin history and only the third in U.S. history. This number of signatures was almost as many as the total votes that elected the Governor to office; moreover, there were sufficient signatures collected to recall the Lt. Governor and four GOP state senators.[17]

- *Ohio pushback against anti-union tactics.* In November 2011, Ohio voters overwhelmingly rejected a restrictive collective bargaining law championed by new Governor John Kasich. By a vote of 61 to 39 percent, voters defeated Issue 2 as a referendum on the law, gaining a victory for some 360,000 public employees in the state. [18]

- *New York hotel workers health care plan.* Over the last 12 years, starting from a small clinic on Manhattan's West Side this plan of New York's Local 6 has grown to five comprehensive health care centers serving some 88,000 hotel workers. Except for a small co-payment for drugs ($5 for generics, $15 for non-generics), there is no cost-sharing. This is a "bottom up" plan to serve its members, starting with a solid primary care base. All physicians are on salary, and the union drives hard agreements with hospitals and other providers. It has been able to effectively contain costs. By comparison, the least expensive private HMO in the area, Healthfirst, is three times as expensive.[19]

- *Single-payer initiatives in Vermont, Hawaii and Montana.* Vermont made some progress toward universal health care for its residents in 2011 with enactment of a health reform bill. While calling health care a public good and declaring that the State has an obligation to assure universal access to "high-quality, medically necessary health services for all Vermonters," the bill fell short of single-payer reform by allowing continued existence of multi-payer financing and tiered care.[20] Efforts are being made, with a supportive Governor in Hawaii, to get a federal waiver and establish single-payer system; the state has an advantage in having a partial ERISA exemption since the 1970s and the Hawaii Medical Association has already passed a resolution supporting single-payer.[21] The Governor of Montana is also planning to pursue a single-payer system that would wrap Medicaid, Medicare, VA and Indian Health Services funding together.[22]

- *Solid majority support of physicians and other health professionals for national health insurance.* A 2008 national study of more than 2,200 U.S. physicians in 13 specialties found that 59 percent support single-payer national health insurance; except for three specialties (surgery, anesthesiology and radiology), more than 50 percent in all of the other specialties favored single-payer.[23]

- ***Shift in conservative publications toward concept of universal coverage.*** We are starting to see more conservative authors and publications very concerned over the directions of markets in this country. Here is one example by John E. Girouard in *Forbes* in 2009:

> "For-profit health insurance has undermined our economy and society. . . . We lost the positive aspects of affiliation health insurance starting in the 1960s and through the 1980s when Wall Street discovered there was money to be made turning nonprofit health insurers, hospitals and nursing homes into investor-owned companies What we got was a massive conflict-of-interest—profit vs. public good—that has culminated in a dysfunctional health delivery system that has undermined our economy, reduced our national wealth and torn our social fabric." [24]

- ***Opposition of small business to Citizens United decision.*** The U.S. Chamber of Commerce is a powerful advocate of Big Business, but in no way speaks for small business in America. A recent survey by Lake Research of three small business organizations—American Sustainable Business Council, the Main Street Alliance and Small Business Majority—found that 88 percent of small business owners have a negative view of the role that money plays in politics.[25]

- ***Powerful backlash by American women to funding cutbacks of Planned Parenthood.*** When the Susan G. Komen for the Cure Foundation attempted to slip through a funding cut of $680 million to Planned Parenthood, an immediate firestorm erupted among women across the country. A massive protest erupted through social media networks (including Facebook and Twitter) that soon led to the resignation of Karen Handel, the high-ranking Komen official seen to be leading the funding cutback. Planned Parenthood has funded breast screenings for low-income women for years. The significance of this event led Katrina vanden Heuvel, editor and publisher of *The Nation,* to observe:

"The episode was a powerful reminder that women are not willing to sit by as their rights are taken away by a hyper-organized band of religious extremists who pressure and intimidate allegedly neutral institutions like Komen. It made clear that anti-choicers aren't the only ones who can throw their weight around. And it enabled Planned Parenthood to collect $3 million to support its vital mission. . . .

If the grassroots energy that brought Komen in line can work similar magic on Congress—by electing pro-choice candidates and keeping up the pressure after the election—then real progress might actually be possible."[26]

- **GOP overreach.** To the extent that Republicans gain strength in the 2012 election cycle, or are blamed by the public for their regressive policies in further decimating the middle class and increasing the ranks of Americans living in poverty, a growing backlash to GOP policies may well improve the odds for major reform of Wall Street, health care and other of our institutions. Based on the performance of GOP presidential candidates in the primary season, a growing part of the electorate is likely to see through their rhetoric and see that Republicans have no real answers for the country's problems. Given these problems, the brazen arrogance of the Republican establishment boggles the mind—the Republican National Committee has recently even proposed that the 105-year old anticorruption ban on direct corporation contributions to candidates and parties be scrapped as unconstitutional![27]

  Republicans may well overreach on their proposed health care policies as well. One good example is the powerful public backlash initiated by womens' health advocates and others over threats to contraception and abortion services. We know that well over 90 percent of women and men (including many Catholics) support contraception. In one instance, Republican Governor Bob McDonnell of Virginia was forced to back down from his initial support of a bill that would have mandated that women undergo transvaginal ultrasound before having an abortion.[28]

- ***Growing recognition among senior economists that our version of capitalism is failing and that we need a New Capitalism.*** Here is what Joseph Stiglitz says on the subject:

"Today the challenge is to create a New Capitalism. We have seen the failures of the old. But to create this New Capitalism will require trust—including trust between Wall Street and the rest of society. Our financial markets have failed us, but we cannot function without them. Our government failed us, but we cannot do without it. The Reagan-Bush agenda of deregulation was based on mistrust of government; the Bush-Obama attempt to rescue us from the failure of deregulation was based on fear. The inequities that have become manifest as wages fall, unemployment rise, but bank bonuses soar, or as corporate welfare is strengthened and the corporate safety net is expanded as that for ordinary citizens is cut back, generate bitterness and anger. An environment of bitterness and anger, of fear and mistrust, is hardly the best one in which to begin the long and hard task of reconstruction. But we have no choice: if we are to restore sustained prosperity, we need a new set of social contracts based on trust between all the elements of our society, between citizens and government, between this generation and the future."[29]

At this writing (April 2012), as the GOP primary election season drones on, and as the candidates agree on reactionary policies including less government, cutback of "entitlements", no tax increases, and protecting the rich, they tend to identify themselves as part of the 1 percent out of touch with the plight of ordinary Americans; (eg. Romney speakers' fees of $374,000 as "not very much"); their rhetoric may appeal to the Tea Party and their social conservative base, but will likely be interpreted by the broad electorate as against the American Dream.

And as the primary GOP campaigns whittle down the presidential field, Obama gains a wide-open opportunity to run as a populist candidate in the general election. Kicking off his 2012 election campaign in a speech evoking the populism of Teddy Roosevelt in Osawatomie, Kansas in December 2011, in an effort to join forces with the 99 percent, this is how he took on the GOP:

> "After all that's happened, after the worst economic crisis, the worst financial crisis since the Great Depression, they [the GOP] want to return to the same practices that got us into this mess. In fact, they want to go back to the same policies that stacked the deck against middle-class Americans for way too many years. And their philosophy is simple: We are better off when everybody is left to fend for themselves and play by their own rules.
> I am here to say they; are wrong. I'm here in Kansas to reaffirm my deep conviction that we're greater together than we are on our own."[30]

But as we all know, it is easier to talk than to walk the walk.

Health Care Reform: Is it Achievable Given Political Will and a Functioning Democracy?

The excesses of the market-based "system" that we have seen *can* be controlled if we are serious about it, and if we can overcome the barriers of corporate governance. And we already know enough from the ineffective experience of incremental reform attempts over the last 30 years to know what will work and what will not work. A logical pathway to real health care reform has been offered in my 2010 book *Hijacked: The Road to Single-Payer in the Aftermath of Stolen Health Care Reform.* (Table 12.2)[31]

The single most important reform of all is to eliminate the private health insurance industry. Despite high levels of government subsidies, it has had a long ride and has failed the public interest. Despite its claims, it offers no value over public financing, and instead drains our system of money that could be better spent on actual health care. As tribal wisdom of the Dakota Indians that has been passed on from generation to generation says: "When you discover that you are riding a dead horse, best strategy is to dismount."

Shifting to single-payer financing based on one risk pool of all 310 million of us will enable other necessary reforms to take place, including assuring access to all Americans to physicians and hospitals

TABLE 12.2

A Nine-Point Approach to Real Health Care Reform

1. Organize for single payer public financing; abandon our multi-payer system dominated by a failing private insurance industry.
2. Demand that policy alternatives be based on credible documented health policy science and experience, not on ideology, wishful thinking, or corporate bottom lines.
3. Recognize that health care resources are limited, and must be stewarded responsibly for care of our entire population.
4. Establish an independent, non-partisan, science-based national commission to evaluate diagnostic and therapeutic interventions for comparative efficacy and cost-effectiveness, with authority to recommend coverage and reimbursement policies.
5. Change how physicians are paid.
6. Rebuild the primary care workforce.
7. Lead so the president will follow.
8. Establish majority rule in the Senate without filibuster blockade.
9. Mobilize popular support for single payer and build a social movement for real health care reform.

of their choice; how physicians, other health professionals, hospitals and other facilities are paid; what services will be provided that are both efficacious and cost-effective; and providing for accountability of the new system. Such a shift, of course, would have to overcome a massive counter attack and disinformation by the dying insurance industry, as noted in Table 12.3 (p. 208).[32]

As a member of a group of activists, Michael Moore and others came up with this helpful proposal, *10 Things We Want*, to the General Assembly of Occupy Wall Street:[33]

"1. Eradicate the Bush tax cuts for the rich and institute new taxes on the wealthiest Americans and on corporations, including a tax on all trading on Wall Street (where they currently pay 0%).

2. Assess a penalty tax on any corporation that moves American jobs to other countries when that company is already making profits in America. Our jobs are the most important national treasure and they cannot be removed from the country simply because someone wants to make more money.

3. Require that all Americans pay the same Social Security tax on all of their earnings (normally, the middle class about 6% of their income to Social Security; someone making $1 million a year pays about 0.6% (or 90% less than the average person). This law would simply make the rich pay the same percentage as what everyone else pays.

4. Reinstate the Glass-Steagall Act, lacing serious regulations on how business is conducted by Wall Street and the banks.

5. Investigate the Crash of 2008, and bring to justice those who committed any crimes.

6. Reorder our nation's spending priorities (including the ending of all foreign wars and their cost of over $2 billion a week). This will re-open libraries, reinstate band and art and civics classes in our schools, fix our roads and bridges and infrastructure, wire the entire country for 21st century internet, and support scientific research that improves our lives.

7. Join the rest of the free world and create a single-payer, free and universal health care system that covers all Americans all the time.

8. Immediately reduce carbon emissions that are destroying our planet and discover ways to live without the oil that will be depleted and gone by the end of this century.

9. Require corporations with more than 10,000 employees to restructure their board of directors so that 50% of its members are elected by the company's workers. We can never have a real democracy as long as most people have no say in what happens at the place they spend most of their time: their job. (Germany has such a law, which has helped it become the world's leading manufacturer).

10. We, the people, must pass three constitutional amendments that will go a long way toward fixing the core problems we now have. These include:

    a) A constitutional amendment that fixes our broken

electoral system by (1) completely removing campaign
contributions from the political process; (2) requiring all
elections to be publicly financed; (3) moving election day
to the weekend to increase voter turnout; (4) making all
Americans registered voters at the moment of their birth;
and (5) banning computerized voting and requiring that
all elections take place on paper ballots.

b) A constitutional amendment declaring that corporations
are not people and do not have the constitutional rights
of citizens. This amendment should also state that the
interests of the general public and society must always
come before the interests of corporations.

c) A constitutional amendment that will act as a "second bill
of rights" as proposed by President Franklin D. Roosevelt:

TABLE 12.3

Everyone Into the Risk Pool: Pros and Cons

Power of the Pool	Benefits	"Fear factor" argument against change
Bulk purchasing power	The bigger the buyer, the cheaper the price	Who wants government in our medicine cabinets? ---------------------------------- Choice of drugs and development of new cures will shrink
Standardized benefits	Security and protection	Lowest common denominator care. Rationing of medical procedures. "Death panels."
One huge network of doctors and hospitals	Choice and affordability	Loss of choice and access to best doctors
Cost controls over doctors, hospitals, and medical providers	Savings mean the health care system can treat more patients	The best doctors won't practice and hospitals will provide shoddy care.

that every American has a human right to employment, to health care, to a free and full education, to breathe clean air, drink clean water and eat safe food, and to be cared for with dignity and respect in their old age."

Much as we will hear from the right that all this would be socialism, it would involve a stronger role of a more efficient government elected through a more transparent and honest process befitting the democracy we claim to be. In health care, public financing would fund a private delivery system in a way that assures the best possible care for all Americans based on medical need (a civilized concept discovered long ago by almost all other industrialized nations!). Such a system would be a win-win for almost all the interests now involved in health care—most importantly patients and their families; health professionals able to spend more time with patient care; hospitals and other facilities that can predict their budgets from year to year; industries on the supply side that can benefit from large markets if they have effective and safe products; and employers that gain a healthier workforce with less expense to them. The only big loser will be the private insurance industry, but it no longer deserves to be kept alive by taxpayer dollars.

As movement toward these kinds of fundamental reforms gain strength, we will see a battle royale from corporate interests defending the status quo. But we're getting close to a collapse of the health care system, as much of the population is already aware. Recall that the average family of four now with an employer-sponsored PPO spends more than $19,000 on health care when annual median household income is only about $49,000, clearly an unsustainable hardship.

Health care, our financial system and our economy are in crisis. We can't do well by trying to keep on muddling through. This country has dealt successfully with other similar crises in the past, and will have to do so again. Bill Moyers brings us this useful historical perspective:[34]

"Take heart from the past and don't ever count the people out. During the last quarter of the 19th century, the industrial revolution created extraordinary wealth at the top and excruciating misery at the bottom. Embattled citizens rose up. Into their hearts, wrote the progressive Kansas journalist William Allen White, 'had come a sense that their civilization needed recast-

ing, that their government had fallen into the hands of self-seek-
ers, that a new relation should be established between the haves
and have-nots.' Not content to wring their hands and cry 'Woe
is us', everyday citizens researched the issues, organized to
educate their neighbors, held rallies, made speeches, petitioned
and canvassed, marched and marched again. They ploughed the
fields and planted the seeds—sometimes in bloody soil—that
twentieth century leaders used to restore 'the general welfare' as
a pillar of American democracy. They laid down the now-endan-
gered markers of a civilized society: legally ordained minimum
wages, child labor laws, workmen's safety and compensation
laws, pure food and safe drugs, Social Security, Medicare and
rules that promote competitive markets over monopolies and
cartels. Remember: Democracy doesn't begin at the top; it be-
gins at the bottom, when flesh-and-blood human beings fight to
rekindle the patriot's dream."

We have plenty to do, so let's get on with it!
And remember what Mahatma Gandhi said about long odds:

"First they ignore you, then they laugh at you, then they fight
you, then you win."

References

1. Krugman, P. America's unlevel playing field. *New York Times,* January 9, 2012:
   A17.
2. Hedges, C. *The World As It Is: Dispatches on the Myth of Human Progress.*
   New York. Nation Books/Truthdig, 2010: p. 13.
3. Lakoff, G, Haas, E, Smith, GW, Parkinson, S. *The Logic of the Health Care
   Debate.* Berkeley, CA: A Rockridge Institute Report, October 15, 2007.
4. Castellanos, A. GOP health care talking points. July 7, 2009. As cited by the
   Washington Post, July 20, 2009.
5. Ibid # 3: pp. 61-2.
6. Geyman, JP. *Do Not Resuscitate: Why the Health Insurance Industry Is Dying
   and How We Must Replace It.* Monroe, Me. Common Courage Press, 2008,
   p.186.
7. Website of Copernicus Healthcare (htpp://www.copernicus-healthcare.org)
8. Menzel, P, Light, DW. A conservative case for universal access to health care.

 Hastings Center Report, July-August 2006, p. 9.
9. Ibid # 6, p. 187.
10. Sanders, B. Letter to supporters, December 2011.
11. Van Gelder, S, Korten, D, Piersanti, S. Ten ways the Occupy movement changes everything. *Truthout*, November 10, 2011.
12. Stone, R. Health care versus wealth care: investors with a conscience should divest from health insurance companies. *Tikkun*, September 16, 2011.
13. Ibid # 12.
14. Healthcare-NOW! Divestment Campaign for Healthcare. Accessed February 14, 2012 at htpp://www.healthcare-now.org/campaigns/divestment/
15. Congressional Budget Office. Long-term analysis of a budget proposal by Chairman Ryan. April 5, 2011.
16. Ferguson, S. Montana State Supreme Court: Citizens United not welcome here. *Truthout*, January 4. 2012.
17. Marley, P, Stein, J, Tolan, T. Democrats file 1 million signatures for Walker recall. *Milwaukee Wisconsin Journal Sentinel*, JSOnline, January 18, 2012.
18. Fields, R. Ohio voters overwhelmingly reject Issue 2, dealing a blow to Gov. John Kasich. *The Plain Dealer*, Cleveland.com, November 8, 2011.
19. Kuttner, R. A model of health. *The American Prospect,* November 7, 2011.
20. Press release. Vermont health law spurs fresh interest in single-payer reform: doctors group. Physicians for a National Health Program. Chicago, IL, May 25, 2011
21. Kemble, SB. Hawaii single-payer update 06-12-11. *Health Care Talk* (HCTalk com), June 12, 2011.
22. Montana pursues single-payer health plan. *The Progressive Populist* 17 (19): 23, November 1, 2011.
23. Carroll, AE, Ackermann, RT. Support for national health insurance among U.S. physicians: Five years later. *Ann Intern Med* 1481: 566-7, 2008.
24. Girouard, JE. The capitalist case for nonprofit health insurance. *Forbes.com*, October 12, 2009.
25. Weissman, R. Editorial. Small business, corporate interests diverge. *Public Citizen News* 32 (1): 3, 2012.
26. Vanden Heuvel, K. Editorial. The Komen omen. *The Nation* 294 (9): 3, February 27, 2012.
27. Editorial. Back to the robber barons. *New York Times*, January 13, 2012:A18.
28. Tavernise, S. Shift in Virginia on abortion bill. *New York Times*, February 23, 2012: A1.
29. Stiglitz, JE. *Freefall: America, Free Markets, and the Sinking of the World Economy*. New York. W. W. Norton & Company, 2010: pp. 208-9.
30. Obama, B. as quoted by Kornacki, S. President Obama: evolution of a populist. *The Progressive Populist* 18 (1):1,8, 2012.
31. Geyman, JP. *Hijacked: The Road to Single Payer in the Aftermath of Stolen Health Care Reform*, Monroe, ME. Common Courage Press, 2010, p. 235.
32. Court, J. *The Progressive's Guide to Raising Hell: How to Win Grassroots Campaigns, Pass Ballot Box Laws, and Get the Change We Voted For.* White

River Junction, VT. Chelsea Green Publishing, 2010, p. 96.

33. Moore, M. Don't sit this one out: What's your vision for Occupy Wall Street? *Truthout*, November 23, 2011.

34. Moyers, B. Out politicians are money launderers in the trafficking of power and policy. Keynote address at the 40th Anniversary of Public Citizen. Washington, D.C., November 2, 2011.

INDEX

About the Author

John Geyman, M.D. is professor pmeritus of family medicine at the University of Washington School of Medicine in Seattle, where he served as Chairman of the Department of Family Medicine from 1976 to 1990. As a family physician with over 25 years in academic medicine, he has also practiced in rural communities for 13 years. He was the founding editor of *The Journal of Family Practice* (1973 to 1990) and the editor of *The Journal of the American Board of Family Practice* from 1990 to 2003. His most recent books are *Health Care in America: Can Our Ailing System Be Healed?* (Butterworth-Heinemann, 2002), *The Corporate Transformation of Health Care: Can the Public Interest Still Be Served?* (Springer Publishing Company, 2004), *Falling Through the Safety Net: Americans Without Health Insurance* (2005), *Shredding the Social Contract: The Privatization of Medicare* (2006), *The Corrosion of Medicine: Can the Profession Reclaim its Moral Legacy?* (2008), *Do Not Resuscitate: Why the Health Insurance Industry is Dying, and How We Must Replace It* (2008), *Hijacked: The Road to Single Payer in the Aftermath of Stolen Health Care Reform* (2010), *Breaking Point: How the Primary Care Crisis Endangers the Lives of Americans* (2011), and *The Cancer Generation: Baby Boomers Facing a Perfect Storm*-Second Edition (2012). Dr. Geyman served as President of Physicians for a National Health Program from 2005 to 2007 and is a member of the Institute of Medicine.

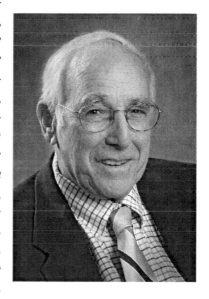